Praises for Apple Cider Vinegar & The Bragg Healthy Lifestyle

These are just a few of the thousands of testimonials we receive yearly, praising The Bragg Health Books for the rejuvenation healthy benefits they reap – physically, mentally and spiritually. We will look forward to hearing from you also.

Thanks to the Bragg Health Books, they were our introduction to healthy living. We are very grateful to you and your father.
– Marilyn Diamond, Co-Author "Fit For Life"

In 1998 I severely broke my left leg and doctors mended it with plates, screws and bolts. I developed staph and pus infections and sores on bottom of my left foot. I had constant pain in my foot, ankle and knee. Since then I have had problems walking up and down stairs and kneeling was impossible. Then I started taking Bragg's Apple Cider Vinegar (2 Tbsps 3x a day). Two days after I started, the soreness in my knees disappeared and climbing the stairs is now pain free and all the other problems are gone!!! I never expected all these results, I give full credit to Bragg's Apple Cider Vinegar. Thank you. – Duke Jones, Oregonia, OH, Retired Police Officer

Bragg ACV is great. The Bragg Vinegar Drink has become our Life Supporting System and we passionately support it and cannot live without it. We thank you for all the many ways we can use your vinegar with the miracle mother enzymes.
– Yasuko and Hiro Hashimoto, CEO of NEC, Japan

When I was a young gymnastics coach at Stanford University, Paul Bragg's words and example inspired me to live a healthy lifestyle. I was twenty-three then; now I'm over sixty, and my health, energy and fitness serves as a living testimonial to Paul Bragg's health wisdom, carried on by his health dedicated crusading daughter, Dr. Patricia Bragg. Thank you both!
– Dan Millman, Author "The Way of the Peaceful Warrior"
www.danmillman.com

Bragg Books were my conversion to the healthy way.
– James F. Balch, M.D.,
Co-Author "Prescription for Nutritional Healing"

The use of Bragg organic apple cider vinegar is a wonderful health aid, the #1 food I recommend in helping to maintain the body's vital acid-alkaline balance. Everyone should read this Bragg Vinegar Book.
– Gabriel Cousens, M.D., Author of *Conscious Eating* and *Spiritual Nutrition*

a

Praises for Apple Cider Vinegar & The Bragg Healthy Lifestyle

Paul Bragg saved my life at age 15 when I attended the Bragg Health Crusade in Oakland. I thank the Bragg Healthy Lifestyle for my long, healthy, active life spreading health and fitness.
– Jack LaLanne, Thankful Bragg follower since 15 years old

Your dad, Dr. Paul Bragg IS the FATHER of the natural health industry and entire natural health movement. Everything that has been done in natural health and physical culture since has been based on the pioneering vision and principles articulated by Dr. Bragg. He gave us all our healthy direction! – Dr. William Wong, Mineral Wells, TX

As a youth I had a learning disability and was told I would never read, write or communicate normally. At 14 I dropped out of school and at 17 ended up in Hawaii surfing. My road to recovery led me to Dr. Paul Bragg who changed my life by giving me one simple affirmation to repeat: "I am a genius and I apply my wisdom." Dr. Bragg inspired me to live a healthy lifestyle and go back to school and get my education and from there miracles happened. I've authored 54 training programs and 14 books and love to crusade around the world thanks to Bragg. – Dr. John Demartini,
Author and Dynamic Crusader (www.drdemartini.com)

For 30 years I've followed The Bragg Healthy Lifestyle - It teaches you how to take control of your health and build a healthy future.
– Mark Victor Hansen, Co-Producer, "Chicken Soup for The Soul Series"

I met Paul Bragg in 1964 at "L" Street Beach in Boston. Both Paul and daughter Patricia are dynamic, energetic and life-changers! They have always been health inspirations to millions around the world, but especially to me! I gave my first lecture with them in April 1964, I was 22, I am over 64 now. Patricia has more energy than any 3 people I know put together and loves traveling the world for Bragg Health Crusades.
– Dr. David Carmos and Dr. Shawn Miller, Co-Authors, La Jolla, CA
You're Never Too Old To Become Young (www.perfecthealthnow.com)

I had a tear duct pus infection for 2 days. I remembered I had a bottle of Bragg's Apple Cider Vinegar and dabbed a little on the tear duct. It stung a little, but it soothed the pain and itching. Now it's gone. No doctor, no medicine! Thank you very much. – Carol Huddleston, Sparta, IL

In Medical School I read Dr. Bragg's Health Books and they changed my thinking and the path of my life. I founded the Omega Institute.
- Steven Rechtschaffen, M.D. (www.eomega.org) *famous since 1977*

Praises for Apple Cider Vinegar & The Bragg Healthy Lifestyle

I have suffered an irritable bowel, colitis, spastic colon, constipation and unnatural painful gas for years. I have been on all kinds of medicine. Nothing worked, until I started taking Bragg's Apple Cider Vinegar. Wow! My problem is gone! Why didn't somebody tell me about this sooner? I now have my life back and can socialize again.
– Fran Covert, Aurora, Colorado

I had 99% blockage in my carotid artery and was scheduled for surgery. I started reading the Bragg Vinegar book and using the vinegar drink!!! My Doctor says my artery is now "zero" blockage and my blood pressure and cholesterol levels are perfect. Huge Miracles! Thank You! – Joseph Gajdosz, NY

I lost 102 lbs. with the Bragg Vinegar Drink and Bragg Healthy Lifestyle. I have kept it off for over 15 years, staying away from white flour, sugar and all the refined foods. Thank you.
– Dee McCaffrey, Chemist & Diet Counselor, Tempe, AZ

In 1975 I was diagnosed with coronary heart disease. I followed the Free Bragg Exercise Classes and Lectures at Fort DeRussy in Waikiki, 6 times a week. Over 31 years have passed and I am going strong and healthy at 84 years young thanks to Bragg Healthy Lifestyle. In 1932 my father had severe hip arthritis and was hardly able to walk. He followed the Paul Bragg Healthy Lifestyle with the vinegar drink and was cured of his arthritis.
– Helen Risk, RN, San Diego, CA

As the world's foremost authority on human memory performance, I tell all my students that one cannot have optimum memory without taking Bragg's Apple Cider Vinegar. I've been taking Bragg's ACV all my life. To have a healthy memory you need a healthy brain and to have a healthy brain you need Bragg's ACV.
– David the "Memory Man," CA

I have recently purchased your books, and have been making Bragg Apple Cider Vinegar drinks for only 2 weeks. WOW!! I can't believe it, I have no more brain fog! I have tried so many other products and remedies, but nothing compares to this. I can't thank you enough for what you have done for me, and others across the USA and the world.
God Bless You! – Heather Hayes, Denver, CO

c

Praises for Apple Cider Vinegar & The Bragg Healthy Lifestyle

How I beat cancer, obesity, diabetes, strep and three herniated disks and excruciating pain? The answer was changing to the Bragg's Healthy Lifestyle and daily having the amazing Bragg Vinegar Drink. It changed and saved my life! I had full recovery and also lost 70 lbs. I received a new life and that is just the beginning because my manhood returned that was lost to diabetes – now that's exciting! On my trip to Honolulu I visited the famous free Bragg Exercise Class at Waikiki Beach. I became so regenerated with a wonderful new viewpoint towards living the Bragg Healthy Lifestyle that I now live in Hawaii. I'm invigorated with new energy for life and living! My new purpose for living is to help others reclaim their health rights! I want the world to join The Bragg Health Crusade. I am deeply thankful to Paul and Patricia for my new healthy life!
– Len Schneider, Honolulu, Hawaii

Thank you Paul and Patricia Bragg for my simple, easy to follow Healthy Lifestyle. You make my days healthy!
– Clint Eastwood, Academy Award Winning Film Producer, Director, Actor and Bragg follower for over 55 years

See more ACV & Bragg Health Teaching Praises on pages 111-117

We get letters daily at our Santa Barbara headquarters. We would love to receive a testimonial letter from you on any blessings, healings and changes you experienced after following The Bragg Healthy Lifestyle and this book. It's all within your grasp to be in top health. By following this book, you can reap more Super Health and a happy, longer vital life! It's never too late to begin. Studies show amazing results that were obtained with people in their 80's and 90's, pages 9, 88-90. Receive miracles with healthy nutrition, fasting and exercise! Don't wait – start now!

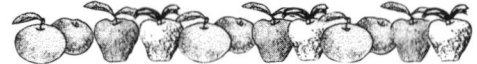

Daily our prayers & love go out to you, your heart, mind & soul.
With Love,

3 John 2   Genesis 6:3

Patricia Bragg

 d   *Miracles can happen every day through guidance and prayer!* – Patricia Bragg

Please enjoy www.bragg.com and follow me on twitter @ patriciabragg

BRAGG
APPLE CIDER VINEGAR
MIRACLE HEALTH SYSTEM

with the

BRAGG HEALTHY LIFESTYLE
**Blueprint for Physical, Mental and Spiritual
Improvement – Healthy, Vital Living to 120**

Genesis 6:3

PAUL C. BRAGG, N.D., Ph.D.
LIFE EXTENSION SPECIALIST
and

PATRICIA BRAGG, N.D., Ph.D.
HEALTH CRUSADER & LIFESTYLE EDUCATOR

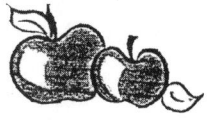

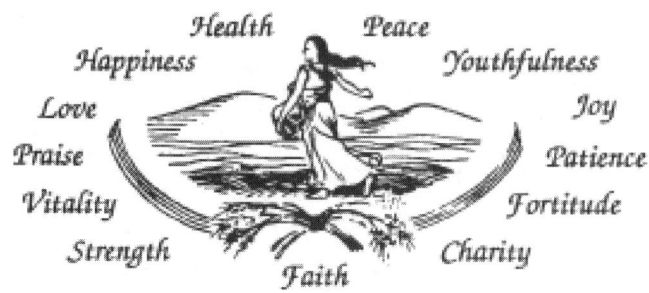

*Health Peace
Happiness Youthfulness
Love Joy
Praise Patience
Vitality Fortitude
Strength Charity
Faith*

BECOME
A Bragg Health Crusader – for a 100% Healthy World for All!

HEALTH SCIENCE
Box 7, Santa Barbara, California 93102 USA

World Wide Web: www.bragg.com

BRAGG

APPLE CIDER VINEGAR

MIRACLE HEALTH SYSTEM

PAUL C. BRAGG, N.D., Ph.D.
LIFE EXTENSION SPECIALIST
and
PATRICIA BRAGG, N.D., Ph.D.
HEALTH CRUSADER & LIFESTYLE EDUCATOR

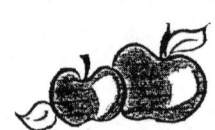
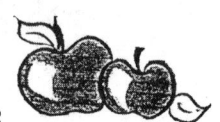

Health Science, Box 7, Santa Barbara, California 93102
Telephone (805) 968-1020, FAX (805) 968-1001
e-mail address: books@bragg.com

Quantity Purchases: Companies, Professional Groups, Churches, Clubs, Fundraisers etc. Please contact our Special Sales Department.

**To see Bragg Books and products on-line,
visit our website: www.bragg.com**

 This book is printed on recycled, acid-free paper,
which saves thousands of trees.

Fifty-seventh Edition MMX
ISBN: 978-0-87790-100-6

Published in the United States
HEALTH SCIENCE, Box 7, Santa Barbara, California 93102 USA

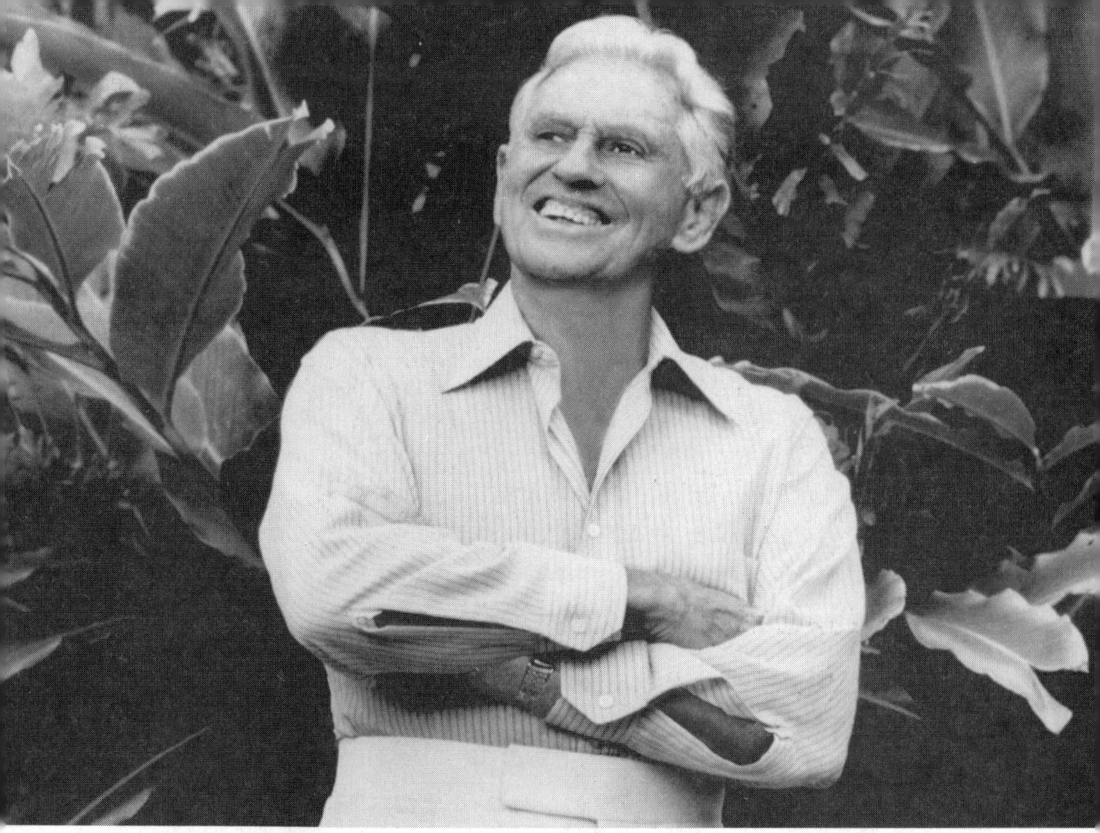

PAUL C. BRAGG, N.D., Ph.D.
World's Leading Healthy Lifestyle Authority

Paul C. Bragg's daughter Patricia and their wonderful, healthy members of the Bragg *Longer Life, Health and Happiness Club* exercise daily on the beautiful Fort DeRussy lawn, at famous Waikiki Beach in Honolulu, Hawaii. View club exercising www.bragg.com. Membership is free and open to everyone to attend any morning – Monday through Saturday, from 9 to 10:30 am – for Bragg Super Power Breathing and Health and Fitness Exercises. On Saturday there are often health lectures on how to live a long, healthy life! The group averages 75 to 125 per day, depending on the season. From December to March it can go up to 150. Its dedicated leaders have been carrying on the class for over 30 years. Thousands have visited the club from around the world and carried the Bragg Health and Fitness Crusade to friends and relatives back home. When you visit Honolulu, Hawaii, Patricia invites you and your friends to join her and the club for wholesome, healthy fellowship. She also recommends visiting the outer Islands (Kauai, Hawaii, Maui, Molokai) for a fulfilling, healthy vacation.

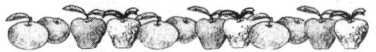

To maintain good health, normal weight and increase the good life of radiant health, joy and happiness, the body must be exercised properly (stretching, walking, jogging, running, biking, swimming, deep breathing, good posture, etc.) and nourished wisely with healthy foods. – Paul C. Bragg

iii

KEEP HEALTHY & YOUTHFUL BIOLOGICALLY WITH EXERCISE & GOOD NUTRITION

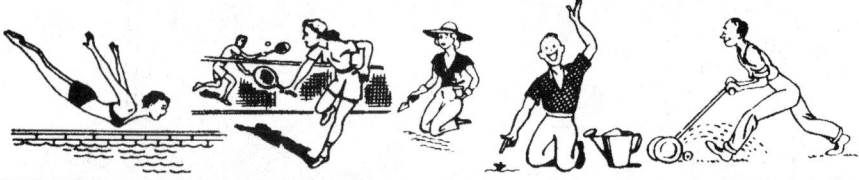

Always remember you have the following important reasons for following The Bragg Healthy Lifestyle:

- The ironclad laws of Mother Nature and God.
- Your common sense, which tells you that you are doing right.
- Your aim to make your health better and your life longer.
- Your resolve to prevent illness so that you may enjoy life.
- Make an art of healthy living; you will be youthful at any age.
- You will retain your faculties and be hale, hearty, active and useful far beyond the ordinary length of years.
- You will also possess superior mental and physical powers!

WANTED – For Robbing Health & Life

KILLER Saturated Fats	CHOKER Hydrogenated Fats
CLOGGER Salt	DEADEYED Devitalized Foods
DOPEY Caffeine	HARD WATER Inorganic Minerals
PLUGGER Frying Pan	JERKY Turbulent Emotions
DEATH-DEALER Drugs	CRAZY Alcohol
GREASY Overweight	SMOKY Tobacco
HOGGY Overeating	LOAFER Laziness

What Wise Men Say

Wisdom does not show itself so much in precept as in life – a firmness of mind and mastery of the appetite. – Seneca

Govern well thy appetite, lest Sin surprise thee, and her black attendant, Death. – Milton

Our prayers should be for a sound mind in a healthy body. – Juvenal

I saw few die of hunger – of eating, a hundred thousand. – Ben Franklin

Your health is your wealth. – Paul C. Bragg

Health is a blessing that money cannot buy. – Izaak Walton

***The natural healing force within us is the greatest force in getting well.*
– Hippocrates, Father of Medicine, 400 BC**

Of all the knowledge, the one most worth having is knowledge about health! The first requisite of a good life is to be a healthy person. – Herbert Spencer

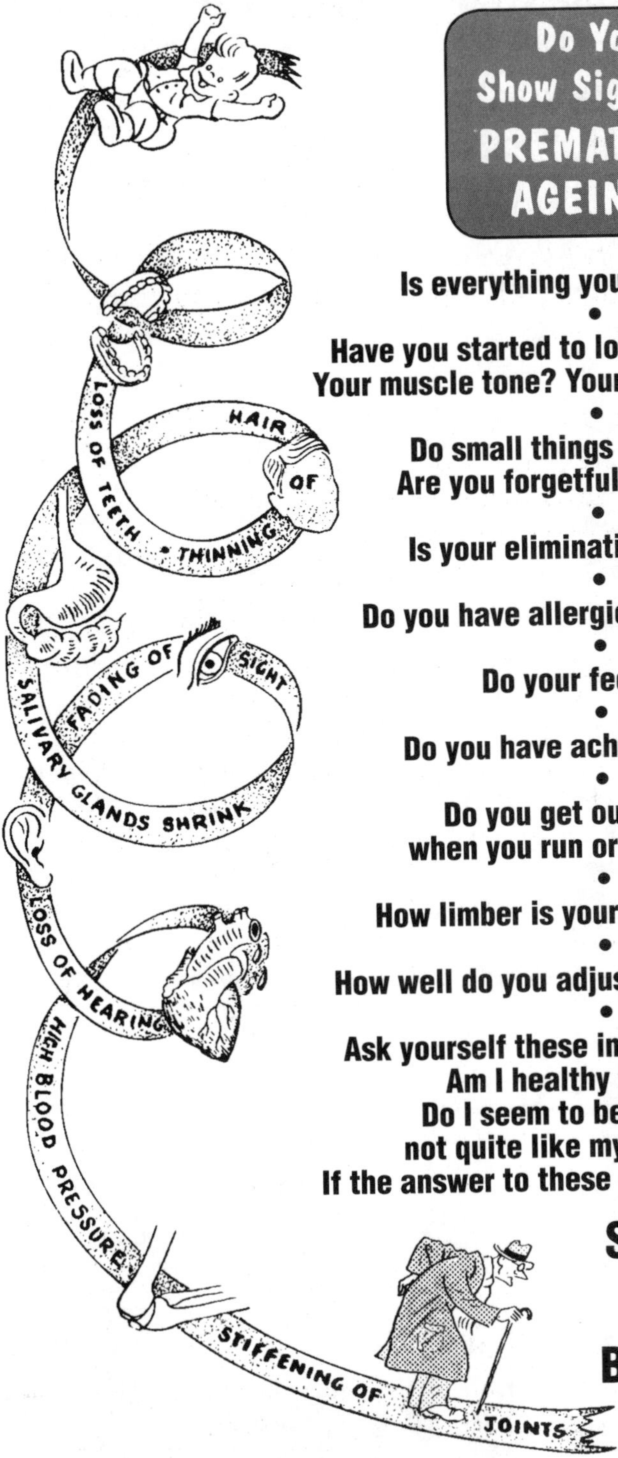

Do You Show Signs of PREMATURE AGEING?

Is everything you do a big effort?

•

Have you started to lose your skin tone?
Your muscle tone? Your energy? Your hair?

•

Do small things irritate you?
Are you forgetful?   Confused?

•

Is your elimination sluggish?

•

Do you have allergies? Joint pains?

•

Do your feet hurt?

•

Do you have aches and pains?

•

Do you get out of breath
when you run or climb stairs?

•

How limber is your back and body?

•

How well do you adjust to cold and heat?

•

Ask yourself these important questions:
Am I healthy and happy?
Do I seem to be slipping and
not quite like myself anymore?
If the answer to these questions are "Yes,"

START TODAY
Living The
Bragg Healthy
Lifestyle!

HAIR OF THINNING

LOSS OF TEETH

FADING OF SIGHT

SALIVARY GLANDS SHRINK

LOSS OF HEARING

HIGH BLOOD PRESSURE

STIFFENING OF JOINTS

He who understands Mother Nature walks with God. .

v

WE NEED YOUR SUPPORT!

With Your Support The Bragg Health Institute Can Continue to Spread Paul C. Bragg's Teachings

For over 80 years we have been sharing Paul C. Bragg's teachings on healthy living worldwide! Millions are following the Bragg Healthy Lifestyle principles and their lives have been changed forever! Everyday people send us letters, e-mails and call, saying – *"Paul Bragg saved my life!"*

Former U.S. Surgeon General, Dr. C. Everett Koop said Paul Bragg did more for the Health of America than anyone person he knew of.

OUR MISSION: To spread health worldwide and inspire youth and people of all ages to achieve optimal health – physically, mentally and spiritually and live long, productive, caring, happy lives.

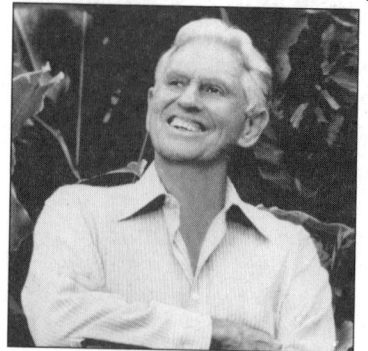

Paul C. Bragg, N.D., Ph.D.
Originator of Health Stores
Life Extension Specialist
Health Crusader to the World

If your life has been touched and helped by Bragg health teachings, please help us carry on the Bragg Legacy into this 21st Century and beyond. Your tax deductible donation to the *Bragg Health Institute* will support our mission to continue the Bragg Message of Health worldwide and inspire future generations.

The non-profit and philanthropic work of the *Bragg Health Institute* funds The *Bragg Health Crusades*, community health, health education lectures, health seminars, and publications on healthy living. The Institute conducts health outreach to youth in schools, organic gardening teaching programs, and helps sponsor health science research and provides scholarships to worthy students pursuing the natural health science professions.

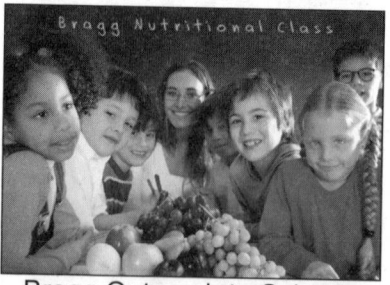

Bragg Outreach to Schools

Please join us in sharing The Bragg Health Legacy!

(Please see page 118 for more information)

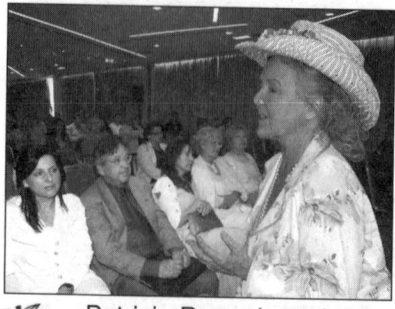

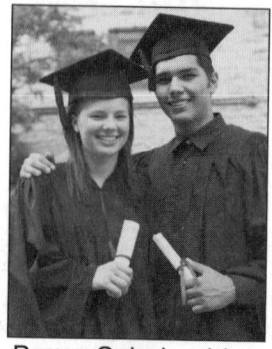

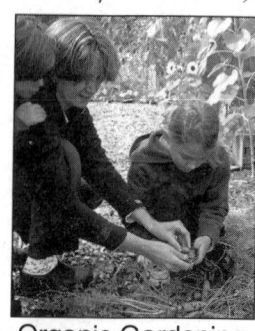

Patricia Bragg lecturing at
Bragg Health Seminars

Bragg Scholarships

Organic Gardening
Teaching Programs

vi

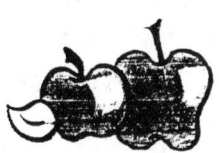

Contents

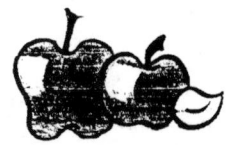

In 400 B.C., Hippocrates, the Father of Medicine, treated his patients with amazing raw Apple Cider Vinegar because he recognized its powerful cleansing and healing qualities. It's a naturally occurring antibiotic and antiseptic that fights germs, viruses, bacteria, even mold.

Title

Nature, time and patience are the three great physicians. – Irish Proverb

"Who satisfieth thy mouth with good things, so that thy youth is renewed like the eagle's." – Psalms 103:5

Happiness is not being pained in body or troubled in mind.
– Thomas Jefferson, Third U.S. President, 1801-1809

Contents

When you sell a man a book you don't just sell him paper, ink and glue, you sell him a whole new life! There's heaven and earth in a real book. The real purpose of books is to inspire the mind to do its own thinking!
– Christopher Morley, Honored American Journalist and Poet

Contents

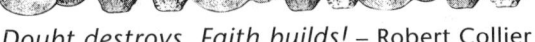

Doubt destroys. Faith builds! – Robert Collier

The natural healing force within us is the greatest force in getting well. – Hippocrates, Father of Medicine, 400 B.C.

You can change and improve the quality of your health by detoxifying your body. Start Your Bragg Healthy Lifestyle today!

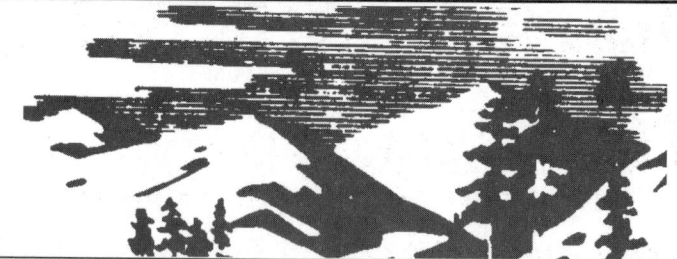

TEN HEALTH COMMANDMENTS

Thou shall respect and protect thy body as the highest manifestation of thy life.

Thou shall abstain from all unnatural, devitalized foods and stimulating beverages.

Thou shall nourish thy body with only natural unprocessed, live foods, that . . .

Thou shall extend thy years in health for loving, sharing with others and charitable service.

Thou shall regenerate thy body by the right balance of activity and rest.

Thou shall purify thy cells, tissue and blood with healthy foods, pure water, clean air and sunshine.

Thou shall abstain from all food when out of sorts in mind or body.

Thou shall keep all thoughts, words and emotions pure, calm, good, loving and uplifting.

Thou shall increase thy knowledge of Nature's Laws, follow them, and enjoy the fruits of thy life's labor.

Thou shall lift up thyself, friends and family by obedience to Mother Nature's and God's Healthy, Natural Laws of Living.

Bragg Healthy Lifestyle Plan

- *Read, plan, plot, and follow through for supreme health and longevity.*
- *Underline, highlight or dog-ear pages as you read important passages.*
- *Organizing your lifestyle helps you identify what's important in your life.*
- *Be faithful to your health goals everyday for a healthy, long, happy life.*
- *Where space allows we include "words of wisdom" from great minds to motivate and inspire you. Please share your favorite sayings with us.*
- *Do write us about your successes following Bragg Healthy Lifestyle & Vinegar Program.*

Patricia Bragg and *Paul C. Bragg*

Open your eyes so you may behold wondrous things out of Thy law. – Psalm 119:18

Bragg
Apple Cider Vinegar
Miracle Health System

How to Use The Powerful Health Qualities of Natural Apple Cider Vinegar

Research worldwide supports and commends what Hippocrates (the father of medicine) found and treated his patients with in 400 B.C. He discovered that natural, undistilled Apple Cider Vinegar (or ACV)* is a powerful cleansing and healing elixir – a naturally occurring antibiotic and antiseptic that fights germs, bacteria, mold and viruses – for a healthier, stronger, longer life!

Versatility of ACV as a powerful body cleansing agent and weight reduction agent is legendary. It's traced to Egyptian urns back to 3000 B.C. The Babylonians used it as a condiment and preservative, while Julius Caesar's army used ACV tonic to stay healthy and fight off disease. The Greeks and Romans kept vinegar vessels for healing and flavoring. It was used in Biblical times as an antiseptic and a healing agent and is mentioned in the Bible. In Paris in the Middle Ages it was sold from barrels by street vendors as a body deodorant, healing tonic and delicious vinegar drink to keep the body healthy and ageless.

Even Christopher Columbus on his voyage to discover America in 1492 had vinegar barrels for prevention of scurvy as did Capt. James Cook on his ships to the South Seas. It helped disinfect and heal the U.S. Civil War soldiers wounds. For centuries in Japan, the feared Samurai warriors drank it for power. The Chinese call vinegar a "friend" because they have used it for centuries to process herbal medicines. ACV has been used for thousands of years not only for health reasons, but as a cleansing agent to remove bacteria, germs, mold, odors, even stains and spots.

A teacher for the day can be a guiding light for a lifetime!
Bragg Books are silent health teachers – never tiring, ready night or day to help you help yourself to health! Our books are written with love and a deep desire to guide you to living a healthy lifestyle. – Patricia Bragg

The best vinegar is organic, raw, unfiltered, unpasteurized apple cider vinegar with the "mother enzyme," available health stores. See back pages for info.

ACV – Mother Nature's Perfect Miracle Food

Natural (undistilled) organic, raw ACV can be called one of Mother Nature's most perfect foods, the worlds first natural medicine. It is made from fresh, crushed apples which are then allowed to mature naturally in wooden barrels to "boost" the natural fermentation. Natural ACV is a rich, brownish color and if held to the light you might see a tiny formation of "cobweb-like" substances we call the miracle "mother". Usually some "mother enzyme" shows at the bottom of the bottle as it ages. It never needs refrigeration! You can also save some "mother" and transfer it to other natural vinegars. When you smell natural ACV, often there is a pungent odor and sometimes it's so ripened it can pucker your mouth and smart your eyes – these are natural, good signs.

Why Has Natural Apple Cider Vinegar Disappeared from Grocers' Shelves?

The blame for the disappearance of natural raw apple cider vinegar from supermarkets lies on the shoulders of the general public, as well as the producers of vinegar. Most people buy food with their eyes, not thinking of good nutrition. Vinegar producers failed to enlighten the public on what powerful health qualities are locked within natural ACV. Why? Because they didn't know the health values of natural, raw, organic, unfiltered, cloudy (to some, less attractive-looking) ACV with the "mother". They produced pasteurized, refined, distilled vinegars because the public preferred it. Filling current supply and demand tragically removed the priceless miraculous "mother" health benefits.

Powerful Health Qualities They Removed

You cannot completely blame the producers of vinegar. They are not nutritionists, nor are they biochemists. Their business is to give the customers what they want. Most people purchase vinegar for flavoring, also for pickling and marinating their foods. Some women use it to rinse their hair after shampooing, as it leaves the hair squeaky clean, softer and much easier to manage.

Organic Apple Cider Vinegar with the "Mother Enzyme" is one of the best body detoxifiers. It can be considered a strong aid to reach the fountain of youth!

ACV Kills Germs, Viruses, Mold & Bacteria

Recent studies show a straight 5% solution of vinegar kills 99% of bacteria, 82% of common mold and 80% of germs & viruses. It's a great germ and virus fighter in homes, kitchens, baths and in hospitals, labs, etc. Some mix it with water to wash windows, as it removes sludge and keeps them sparkling clean, as it does for the body. ACV has hundreds of uses and its versatility is legendary as a powerful household cleansing and deodorizing agent, free of dangerous chemicals. (See cleaning hints – pages 103 to 105.)

ACV Has Proven Powerful Health Qualities

The healthy miracle nutrients that live in the "mother" substance of organic, unfiltered, fully ripened ACV have proven powerful health benefits! Sadly, commercial producers distill their vinegar to meet consumer demand that vinegar be clear. In distilling, the vinegar is turned to steam by heating. Therefore it destroys the powerful "mother enzymes" and distills out life-giving minerals such as potassium, phosphorus, natural organic sodium, magnesium, sulphur, iron, copper, natural organic fluorine, silicon, trace minerals, essential amino acids and many other powerful nutrients including pectin, a fiber that helps reduce bad cholesterol and helps regulate blood pressure. ACV also helps extract calcium from fruits and vegetables, helping to maintain strong bones. Distilling also destroys the natural malic and tartaric acids which are important in fighting body toxins and inhibiting unfriendly bacteria.

ACV is also loaded with potassium. Studies have shown potassium helps prevent hair loss, brittle teeth and nails, sinusitis, runny nose, toxic waste in the body, plus stunted growth! The beta-carotene in ACV helps fight harmful free radicals and breaks down unwanted fat to aid in weight management. ACV also contains malic acid, which relieves fungal and bacterial infections, as well as dissolves the uric acid deposits that form around your aching joints. (See pages 30-31)

Other incredible benefits of ACV are the relief of constipation, headaches, arthritis, indigestion, diarrhea, eczema, sore eyes, chronic fatigue, mild food poisoning, as well as high blood pressure and heartburn symptoms.

Commercial Vinegars are Real Tragedies

Then came the real tragedy: a food chemist produced an imitation vinegar from coal tar! It looked clean, white and tasted like vinegar. Today it's the most popular vinegar in supermarkets. It's cheaper than distilled vinegar or malt vinegar. Most people buy these worthless vinegars. There's nothing good about commercial vinegars, except they look clean and taste like vinegar. They have no health value! They don't contain the health values of organic, raw ACV with the *mother*. Sad fact: millions worldwide never get the health benefits of this natural organic apple cider vinegar as wise Doctor Hippocrates used in 400 B.C.

Millions Suffer from Malnutrition

"Mal" means bad. As a consequence of not getting natural, healthy, balanced diets, millions worldwide suffer from many forms of subclinical malnutrition. This means many people, due to vitamin and mineral deficiencies, feel half-sick most of the time! They lack vim, vigor and "Go Power" and feel tired most of the time. Their daily food intake and the commercial vinegars they use don't provide sufficient vitamins and minerals, nor the potassium their bodies require. They lack vital power and feel exhausted. This is the reason people turn to stimulants like coffee, America's most popular unhealthy drink, and to colas, alcohol, cigarettes and over-the-counter "fix-all" drugs. After these stimulants' effects wear off, they feel terrible. They just exist, and are not living happy, healthy lives!

Coffee – America's #1 Drug Addiction

Coffee drinking (caffeine) is the #1 drug addiction in America! Millions of pounds of coffee are sold to America yearly. That's not to mention the caffeine in soft drinks. Plus there's millions of addicted chocoholics who are hooked on chocolate and sugar – a harmful combination. The shocking list of caffeine-related side effects include: high blood pressure, hypertension, arrythmia, elevated cholesterol, glucose, increased tendencies to allergies, chronic fatigue and autoimmune disorders, etc.

Man is fully responsible for his nature, choices and lifestyle. – Jean-Paul Sartre

You see these unhappy people about you every day. They are washed out and ageing prematurely. Many lack skin and muscle tone and have dark circles and puffy (water) bags under their eyes. Their eyes lose the sparkle of health and youthfulness and become like dead fish eyes. Malnourished people are mostly lifeless and everything they do requires a tremendous effort. They are not really living and most are not happy. Many suffer from depression and mental fatigue – nerve burnout.

One of the great benefits of ACV is that it detoxifies both the bloodstream and various organs of the body. ACV acts as a purifier, breaking down fatty mucous and phlegm. It also prevents your urine from becoming excessively alkaline, assisting your vital organs – kidneys, bladder and liver. ACV also helps promote healthy blood flow to your heart, brain and entire body.

Apples Are Rich in Potassium & Enzymes

"An apple a day keeps the doctor away" is a familiar saying to millions. It carries good common sense. The apple is one of God's great health-giving foods. Apples contain enzymes, boron, iron, minerals, trace minerals, pectin-soluble fiber and a good source of potassium, which is to the soft body tissues as calcium is to the bones and harder tissues. Potassium is the mineral of youthfulness; it is the "artery softener," keeping the arteries of the body flexible and resilient. It's a fighter of dangerous bacteria, viruses and helps dissolve fat. Yes, when you say, "An apple a day keeps the doctor away," this is good, down-to-earth old-fashioned folk medicine for vibrant, life-long health! Since the Garden of Eden the apple has played a vital part in our destiny. People have been eating apples for thousands of years. Apple eaters have a certain healthfulness that non-apple eaters never achieve.

Apples are delicious fruits that most people enjoy eating, but we look on the healthy apple as more than something good to eat. Potassium is the key mineral in the constellation of minerals; it's so important to every living thing that without it there would be no life! Most humans are potassium deficient (page 15) and it reflects in their cell tissues and throughout their entire body. Look around you. How many people do you see that have the super apple glow of health?

There is no wealth greater than the health of the body. – The Bible

Millions Suffer From Potassium Deficiency

Millions living in today's civilization and eating its commercialized, processed foods have a potassium deficiency. The skin and muscle tone are bad. The flesh does not cling firmly to the body's bony framework. Lines and wrinkles fill the face and neck.

One sign is flabby, excess skin hanging over the eyes. If the potassium deficiency continues, the prolapsing eyelids progress. Soon, people are looking out of little slits instead of wide-open eyes. Thousands have turned to eyelid surgery to correct droopy eyelids, also called hooded eyelids, that roll down and rest on their eyelashes causing eyestrain, headaches, etc. If an eye doctor suggests corrective surgery for this, the insurance company usually honors the claim. It's an in/out local procedure. It's wise to have a board certified eye surgeon. People wrongly blame their age for their droopy eyelids, skin changes and lack of muscle tone.

But the truth is . . . you must have potassium to build and maintain youthful, healthy tissues! If you don't get required amount of potassium daily, you soon acquire an old-age look and feel. This premature ageing is usually due to potassium deficiency and unhealthy living!

It is the same in your flower and vegetable garden. Potassium is necessary for the health production of the substances that give rigidity to plant stems and increase their resistance to the many diseases that attack plants. Potassium is also the powerful element that changes seeds into plants and beautiful flowers by progressive development. If plants become deficient in potassium, they stop their growth. If the potassium deficiency is not corrected, the plant slowly starts to wither, turns yellow and dies! The same is true of animals and humans with a potassium deficiency: there is a slow degeneration leading to death of the cells, then death of life.

Every day the average heart, your best friend, beats 100,000 times and pumps 2,000 gallons of blood for nourishing your body. In about 70 years that adds up to more than 360 million (faithful) heartbeats. Please be good to your heart and live The Bragg Healthy Lifestyle for a long, happy, healthy life! Here's to Genesis 6:3 for you. – Patricia Bragg

Refined Foods & Flours Remove Vital Potassium which Causes Poor Health!

Robbed grains: The miller refines and processes our grains to get white flour that will keep for years . . . that becomes the staff of death! Even bugs have more sense – they won't eat it because it has been robbed of its potassium and vital life-giving qualities!

Shocking loss of potassium and nutrients in making white flour: In milling wheat, the miller refines out 25 important food elements, including vital amino acids, vitamin E, bran, the rich B-complex vitamins and potassium. Cows fed refined grain, with the potassium milled out and de-germed, die early of heart failure.

The more they refine vital potassium out of foods, the sicker Americans get: People waste money, time, and energy and suffer the loss of health by being sick. The #1 health plan should be to teach Americans how to live a healthy lifestyle that maintains health by correct eating and living habits. Healthy nutrition will create bones that last a lifetime, cells that resist disease and arteries that stay healthy, cholesterol-free and unclogged!

Bad Nutrition – #1 Cause of Sickness

"Diet-related diseases account for 68% of all deaths."
– Dr. C. Everett Koop

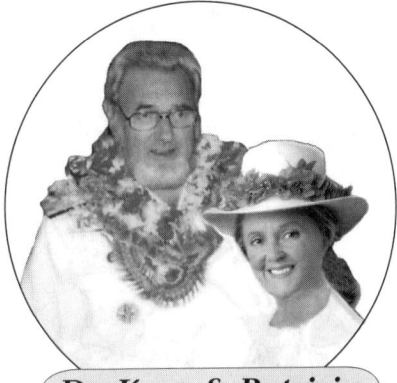

Dr. Koop & Patricia

America's former Surgeon General and our friend, said this in his famous 1988 landmark report on nutrition and health in America. People don't die of infectious conditions as such, but of malnutrition that allows the germs to get a foothold in sickly bodies. Also, bad nutrition is usually the main cause of noninfectious, fatal or degenerative conditions. When the body has its full vitamin and mineral quota, including precious potassium, it's almost impossible for germs to get a foothold in a healthy, powerful bloodstream and tissues!

The Body Has the Seed of Eternal Life

Outside of fatal accidents, there is no reason why a person should leave before his or her time. It has been proven by some of the greatest scientific minds that there are no special diseases of old age. A person should not die simply because they live to 60, 70, 80 or 90 years of age, because calendar age is not toxic. People create their toxins by their eating and living habits.

Most people die of some fatal condition that they have built into their bodies by incorrect living or by violating the natural laws that govern the physical body.

The two great enemies of life are toxic poisons (found in some foods, air, water and soil) and the nutritional deficiencies caused by unhealthy diet. The best prevention of sickness is to eat vital, healthy foods (organic is best and safer), especially those high in potassium. These provide the body with correct, life-giving nourishment.

Every 90 days a new bloodstream, the river of life, is built in the body by the foods you eat, the liquids you drink and the air you breathe. From the bloodstream the body's cells are made, nourished and maintained. Every 11 months we have a new set of billions of miraculous body cells, and every 2 years we have an entirely new set of bones and hard tissues. There is no reason to get old because the body is constantly cleansing and renewing its cells to keep your precious human temple healthy for a long, fulfilled, happy life!

Nutrition directly affects growth, development, reproduction and well-being of an individual's physical and mental condition. Health depends upon nutrition more than on any other single factor. – Dr. William H. Sebrell, Jr.

Laws of health are inexorable; we see people going down and out in their prime of life because no attention is paid to them! – Paul Bragg

Age does not depend upon years, but upon temperament and health.

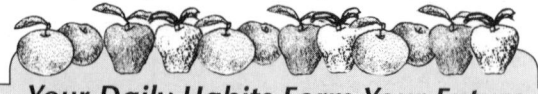

Your Daily Habits Form Your Future

Habits can be wrong, good or bad, healthy or unhealthy, rewarding or unrewarding. The right or wrong habits, decisions, actions, words or deeds . . . are up to you! Wisely choose your habits, as they can make or break your life! – Patricia Bragg

Exercise and ACV Helps Keep You More Youthful, Healthier, Stronger, Flexible and Trim

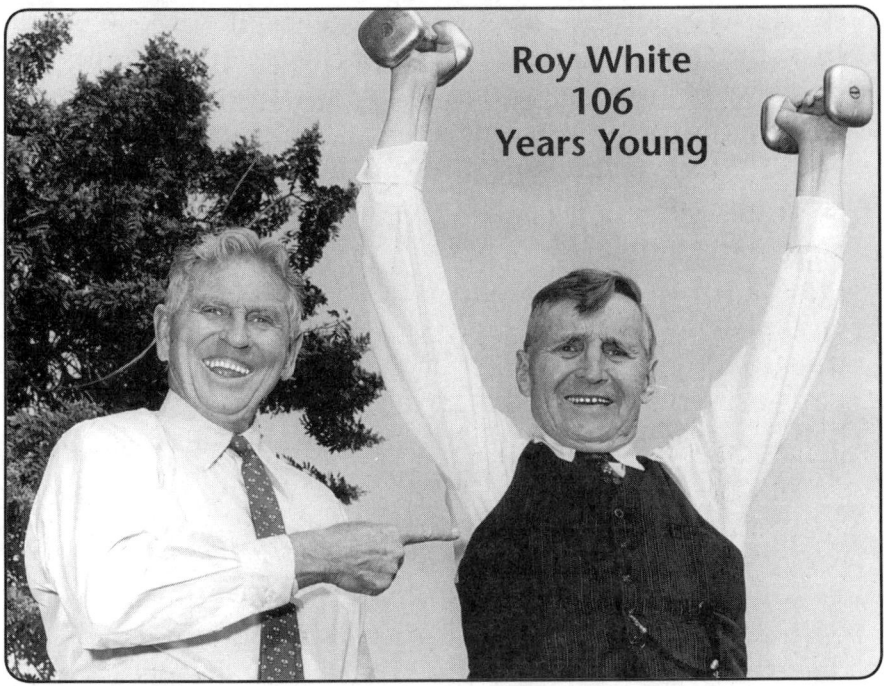

Roy White
106
Years Young

Paul C. Bragg & His Weight Lifting Health Follower, Roy White

Paul and Roy practiced progressive weight training 3 times a week to stay healthy and fit. Scientists have proven that weight training works miracles for all ages by maintaining more flexibility, energy and youthful stamina!

See pages 88-90 for some of the amazing scientific data coming in from around the world on the important longevity, health, renewing and rewarding benefits of regular exercise and living a healthy lifestyle!

Thank you for your wealth of health information in the Bragg Books. I have followed a vegetarian diet and your lifestyle for 31 years. It works! I teach school and summers still lifeguard for the Kentucky Dept. of Parks. I still swim a mile a day! Thank you and may God continue to bless your health outreach!
– Steve House, London, Kentucky

Never shatter someone else's dreams or hopes;
these are as precious, and as rare as life itself.

Man is the sole and absolute master of his own fate forever. What he has sown in the times of his ignorance, he must inevitably reap; when he attains enlightenment, it is for him to sow what he chooses and reap accordingly. – Geraldine Coster

---

Change your mind and change your life.

Dream big, think big, but enjoy the small miracles of everyday life!

Dr. Carrel's Eternal Life Successful Study

Nobel Scientist Dr. Alexis Carrel of the Rockefeller Institute in New York in 1912 kept the cells of an embryo chicken heart alive and healthy for over 35 years by daily monitoring its complete nutrition, cleansing and elimination. A chicken's lifespan averages 7 years!

Apple cider vinegar was given to the chicken embryo daily for its full quota of potassium. Dr. Carrel definitively proved to the entire world that the body has a seed of eternal life. He could have continued this experiment indefinitely to give the embryo immortality, but felt 35 years proved the point that man kills himself by his wrong habits of overeating and living an unhealthy lifestyle. This study showed us the importance of nutrition, cleansing and apple cider vinegar to life, health and longevity! Web: *nobel prize.org/nobel_prizes/medicine/laureates/1912/carrel-bio.html*

 Recently a remarkable study on longevity was done with earthworms. By monitoring their food intake, then decreasing it to only what was nutritionally necessary, these worms multiplied their lifespan (bottom page 55). The results from these and many other studies have revealed the key to longer life. Many scientists know no reason why these same principles could not apply to everyone. Even today the Hunzas of Kashmir and the Georgians of Russia lead active lives to 120 and older!

Potassium Deficiency Can Stunt Growth and Shorten Lifespan

We have enjoyed making over 10 scientific health expeditions throughout the world, studying the health, longevity and growth of various races of people. We found areas where the topsoil was deficient in potassium and the people living off foods grown from this potassium-deficient soil were prone to be stunted in growth and have a shorter lifespan. The pygmies of Africa are stunted and short-lived. The same is true of the Arctic Eskimos. In their daily diet, they just do not get the required amount of potassium and other minerals that are so important to growth, health and long life.

The strongest principle of growth lies in the human choice. – George Elliot

Mentally Handicapped Children and Adults Suffer from Potassium Deficiency

We have closely studied the relationship between mentally handicapped children and adults and potassium deficiency. Many years ago, my dad brought 3 children to our home for study and observation. Three times daily – morning, noon and night – the children had the ACV drink (1 tsp. ACV and 1 tsp. raw honey, both rich in potassium, in glass of distilled water). Dad put the children on The Bragg Healthy Lifestyle which gave them extra amounts of potassium. Daily they were given multiple vitamin-mineral supplements and regular niacin (50 mgs – vitamin B-3). In 3 weeks, these children became more mentally alert. After living in our home for less than a year, they were able to resume their schooling with children their own age!

Another amazing study – we brought three mentally handicapped adults into our home. After putting them on the ACV routine plus living The Bragg Healthy Lifestyle, they became self-supporting in less than a year!

Potassium Deficiency Produces Senility

Throughout the world, there are millions of senile, prematurely old people. Many don't know their own names, nor can they recognize their family or closest friends. They are just barely existing. It might seem that they have degenerated so much that it's almost a hopeless task to try to save them, but please try! We feel they can be restored to useful lives if the toxic poisons are flushed from their bodies and their nutritional deficiencies (nutrients, potassium pg. 15, and niacin, etc.) are corrected!

Fighting Diabetes with ACV

Taking ACV before a meal is beneficial to people with diabetes. Over 41 million Americans are pre-diabetic and 1 in 5 people currently have diabetes. Recent studies show taking 1-2 tsps. of ACV before meals is proven to dramatically reduce insulin and glucose spikes in the blood. These spikes can also cause Heart Disease in people with Type 2 Diabetes!

I was a diabetic and my blood sugar was out of whack for a year. I was desperate and read about your ACV drink. I tried it! Now my blood sugar is normal. I am astounded and amazed. – Don Hess, Quincy, IL

Miracles with Potassium

Years ago, we selected four senile people we felt could be helped. We put them on The Bragg Healthy Lifestyle with the ACV drink and healthy foods rich in potassium. Out of the four, we were able to save three of them. All three left the convalescent home where they had been confined and became healthy, happy and self-sufficient. Two of them made remarkable recoveries. One went back to contracting and building at 83, and the other in his mid 80s resumed his accounting career!

Most senile people suffer from a clogged arterial system. Potassium is to the soft tissues of the body as calcium is to the hard structures. The potassium goes into the clogged, caked arteries and cleans out the rust and dirt just like vinegar water removes grime from windows (page 105). One can't think clearly if arteries are heavily clogged with cholesterol and toxic poisons.

Potassium might be called the great detergent of the arteries. Potassium slows down the hardening and clogging processes that cause deadly harm to the whole cardiovascular system. Organic, raw ACV contains the miraculous potassium that makes the flesh of farm animals healthier and more tender. There is very little doubt, in animal and man, that the main function of potassium is to keep the tissues healthy, soft and pliable, and to help prevent heart attacks and strokes!

Paul Bragg Talks about Vinegar Miracles on His Family's Farm in His Youth

Long years of research have proven to me that natural apple cider vinegar is a potent source of potassium. I was raised on a large farm. On this farm, we grew many varieties of apples. I was a great apple eater. Each year my father made natural apple cider vinegar and stored it in wooden barrels. On our table we used this natural apple cider vinegar and our large family loved it.

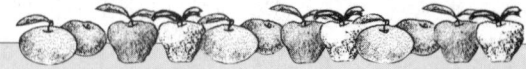

Potassium is the key mineral in the constellation of minerals; it's so important to every living thing that without it there would be no life. Bragg's Organic Raw Apple Cider Vinegar is a rich source of potassium.

ACV Relieves Chronic Fatigue

My father was a splendid farmer and many times I would watch him add ACV to the feed and water of ailing animals (cattle, horses, sheep, dogs, cats, birds, etc.) and it acted like magic. ACV seemed to possess a miracle ingredient that helped restore health to the animals.*

The nearest doctor was 32 miles from our home. If a doctor was needed, he had to come by horse and buggy over miles of rough, dirt roads. So, at our home we developed simple self-health remedies and apple cider vinegar played an important health role.

I remember when my father would put in long hours at the farm during the harvest period. He was up long before daybreak and didn't retire until late at night. I would watch him come into the kitchen, put 2 heaping tsps. of honey in a glass, add 2 tsps. of raw apple cider vinegar, fill the glass with water and then sip it slowly.

I would ask, "Father, why do you drink apple cider vinegar, honey and water?" Father would reply, "Son, farm work is long, hard work. It can produce extreme body fatigue. Whatever is in this apple cider vinegar and honey drink relieves me of that chronic fatigue."

Father was definitely correct. There was an ingredient in that drink that renewed his vitality and relieved him of the chronic fatigue and stiffness. That ingredient was potassium, along with the powerful enzymes, minerals and trace elements that are in organic, raw apple cider vinegar.

Most people today, when they work hard, turn to all kinds of dangerous stimulants to relieve their chronic fatigue: alcohol, tea, coffee, cola drinks and pep pills and other dangerous, addictive drugs.

My father's good advice fell on youthful ears. It was some years later that I realized that my father was a smart man in using raw honey and raw apple cider vinegar, rich in potassium, to combat chronic fatigue.

*ACV also helps animals stay healthy. *Mixture:* 1 cup ACV with 3 cups purified water. Once daily in feed or water: for small animals add 1 tsp. ACV mixture; for large animals add 2 to 3 tsps. Or administer orally with eye dropper, baster or squeeze bottle. To relieve skin rashes or itching apply topically. Add to bath or rinse water to keep skin healthy and ward off fleas. (We have had testimonials of praise in various horse and dog magazines.)

Unhealthy Diet Brings Sickness

At 12, I was sent from my rugged farm life to an expensive military academy as a gift for saving a wealthy man from drowning. That institution's food gradually broke my health! The unhealthy diet of sugared, refined, overcooked and dead foods served there ruined my health. It made me the victim of a consuming disease, tuberculosis.

At no time did I see our wonderful ACV or raw honey at the table of the military academy. It was not until I met the great healer Dr. Rollier at his health sanitarium in Switzerland, where I regained my health, that I again came in contact with the miracles of ACV and *honey, both rich in essential potassium! I owe much of my recovery to apple cider vinegar and honey, as they are persistent fighters against germs and toxins! Each morning, I was given the same drink my father took for energy and health. Dr. Rollier urged us to put apple cider vinegar on all of our raw vegetable salads and steamed greens. He also urged us to eat an abundance of raw vegetables and fresh fruits each day as they are Mother Nature's purifiers. He was a wise natural health minded doctor and knew how valuable potassium and raw fruits and vegetables are for maintaining 100% health.

14

I was 100% cured from TB in less than 2 years after cleansing and rebuilding myself with a balanced natural diet, correct deep breathing, exercise and Alpine sunshine. Healthy living was my cure! I have been an ardent user of organic, raw ACV and raw honey ever since. In our Bragg health teachings and writings we have always advocated the use of this miraculous source of potassium.

It was in Switzerland that I started to fulfill my earlier pledge to God, that if I recovered my health, I would become a health crusader and devote my life to sharing the message of health and wellness with the world! When I finished my schooling, I went on to full-time crusading for a healthier world! (See the Bragg Bio back pages.)

Raw honey has miraculous nutrients (vitamins, potassium, enzymes, etc.). It's a natural occurring antibiotic & antiseptic. Ancient Egyptian medicine touted honey as an essential natural cure-all, listing 500 honey remedies. Hippocrates, father of medicine, prescribed honey as it fights bacteria & ulcers, blocks infection, combats inflammation, reduces pain, improves circulation, stimulates regrowth of tissue, makes healing faster & reduces scarring. ACV & honey together are nature's perfect cure! www.rawhoneybest.com

Body Signs of Potassium Deficiency

🍎 *Bone and muscle aches and pains, especially lower back.*

🍎 *The body feels heavy, tired and it's an effort to move.*

🍎 *Shooting pains when straightening up after leaning over.*

🍎 *Dizziness upon straightening up after leaning over.*

🍎 *Morning dull headaches upon arising and when stressed.*

🍎 *Dull, faded-looking hair that lacks sheen and luster.*

🍎 *The scalp is itchy and dry. Dandruff, premature hair thinning or balding may occur.*

🍎 *The hair is unmanageable, mats, often looks straw-like, and is sometimes extremely dry and other times oily.*

🍎 *The eyes itch, feel sore and uncomfortable and appear bloodshot and watery. Also, eyelids may be granulated with white matter.*

🍎 *The eyes tire easily and will not focus as they should.*

🍎 *You tire physically and mentally with the slightest effort.*

🍎 *Loss of mental alertness and onset of confusion, making decisions difficult. The memory fails, making you forget familiar names and places you should easily remember.*

🍎 *You become easily irritable and impatient with family, friends and loved ones and even with your business and social acquaintances.*

🍎 *You feel nervous, depressed, in a mental fog, and have difficulty getting things done due to mental and muscle fatigue. Even the slightest effort can leave you exhausted, upset and trembling.*

🍎 *At times, your hands and feet get chilled, even in warm weather, which is a sign of potassium deficiency.*

15

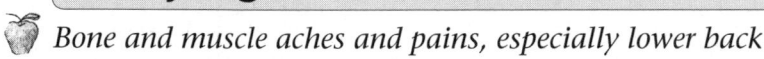

***Potassium deficiency is a proven contributing cause of many illnesses, including:** Arthritis, kidney stones, atrial fibrillation, adrenal insufficiency, celiac disease, high blood pressure, coronary artery disease, ulcerative colitis, hypothyroidism, irritable bowel syndrome, Alzheimer's disease, multiple sclerosis, myasthenia gravis, Crohn's disease, lupus, atherosclerosis, diabetes and stroke.*
– Linda Page, N.D., Ph.D. ***Healthy Healing** (visit her website: www.healthyhealing.com)*

Health Crusader Paul C. Bragg says . . . Life is Thrilling When You Can Help Others!

I founded the health movement and originated, named and started the first Health Food Store. Then, through The Bragg Health Crusades, I inspired hundreds of Bragg students to open the first Health Food Stores in their areas across America and then worldwide. It's thrilling and rewarding to live a life of service helping and inspiring others to live a healthy lifestyle! God has blessed me!

Apple Cider Vinegar Miracle for Overweight

More than a third of Americans are trying to lose weight. Over forty billion dollars are spent yearly on diet programs and products. Rather than a yo-yo diet, these people need The Bragg Healthy Lifestyle and ACV! Please understand ACV will not reduce a person who doesn't control their food intake. But the ACV drink and a healthy diet of 1,200 calories daily, plus regular exercise will do miracles in reducing excess weight*. Take this fat flushing ACV drink 3 times daily (pg. 96). Also the Diet Research Center in England reported this: *"better reducing and firming with ACV daily massage (mix 3 parts Bragg Organic ACV to 1 part Bragg Organic Olive Oil) helps the body reduce fat and cellulite."*

Along with this healthy ACV drink, there must be a healthy reducing diet. (Read the Bragg *Miracle of Fasting* book for more reducing info.) This means that all refined, processed, sugared products and beverages and dairy products are eliminated from your diet (page 86). The diet should consist of a wide variety of fresh organic fruits & vegetables; raw salads & sprouts; raw nuts and seeds; raw, steamed, baked and stir-fried vegetables; brown rice; tofu; beans; and whole grain pastas.

Thermogenic herbs suppress appetite – barley green, spirulina, alfalfa, kelp, sea vegetables, green drinks, etc. – Also take on empty stomach before bed and early am 500 mg L-Carnitine and 200-400 mcg Chromium Picolinate to promote weight loss and firming. Portion control meals, ACV drink, fasting, exercise and these herbs can also help.

*Fat Flushing raw apple cider vinegar burns fat with its acetic acid that helps boost metabolism and dissolve fats, preventing them from being stored as fat and also helps lower blood sugar. You will be less hungry and less bloated.
– Ann Louise Gittleman, Ph.D.

A recent study showed people with large waistlines had shorter lifespans.

Combating Underweight

Apple cider vinegar is proving to be one of the greatest aids to health known to science. It's a 100% natural substance produced by powerful natural enzymes from healthy organic apples, free of any toxic chemicals.

The underweight person is usually deficient in these powerful enzymes and therefore cannot use or burn up the food that is put into their body. No matter how much fatty food, protein or any other kind of food is ingested, often it is not used properly by the body if important enzymes are missing. Enzyme deficiencies always cause problems! If underweight, drink the following ACV cocktail each morning upon arising: 2 tsps. ACV and 2 tsps. honey in a glass of distilled water. Add to this 2 drops of liquid iodine made from seaweed, available in Health Stores. This adds natural iodine, important to body health and helps normalize body weight up or down as needed. Then, with each meal take a multi-digestive enzyme (page 87) and always be faithful to The Bragg Healthy Lifestyle. Remember, healthy foods are needed body fuel to enjoy a healthy long, fulfilled life.

Purify Your Cells by Ridding The Body of Dangerous Toxic Wastes

Toxic poisons are the cause of most troubles in the human body. Most people do not have sufficient vital force to supply the eliminative organs with the strength to remove normal waste from the body. The toxins remain and lodge in the joints and organs of the body. We have a name for each symptom that gives us pain and trouble. Certain toxic wastes that are harmful to the whole body are rendered harmless by a miraculous substance in organic, raw ACV with the powerful *mother enzymes*. Scientists call this protective action *acetolysis*.

In 400 B.C., Hippocrates, the Father of Medicine, treated his patients with amazing raw Apple Cider Vinegar because he recognized its powerful cleansing and miracle healing qualities. It is a naturally occurring antibiotic and antiseptic that fights germs, viruses, bacteria and body toxins.

Through his contact with country medicine as practice for 300 years in Vermont, our friend, Dr. D.C. Jarvis stated that potassium in its natural combination with other trace minerals is so essential to the metabolic process in every form of life on Earth, that without it there would be no life! Taking ACV promotes a potassium-rich blood chemistry to help keep the body tissues soft, pliable and helps prevent hardening of the arteries.

Apple Cider Vinegar for Body Purification

It's time for life changes when you feel badly and don't seem to have the Human Go Power and Vital Force to do the things in life that are necessary! It's time to flush out the energy depleting, problem causing toxic wastes that are clogging your machinery and organs of elimination! Waste products broken down by this ACV process are flushed out. Remember, your important organs of elimination are the bowel, the lungs, the skin and the kidneys. They are your faithful servants! They work hard 24 hours a day to detox and flush out toxic wastes. Many times these eliminative organs need help and that is when the ACV drink comes to their aid!

Follow the ACV daily program. In addition, add 1 tsp. ACV to 6 ounces of salt-free tomato or fresh vegetable juice (carrot and greens) and drink between meals, daily. Be sure to do a cleansing fast 1 day weekly (page 58) and faithfully follow The Bragg Healthy Lifestyle, which is explained throughout the book in full, simple details.

18

Apple Cider Vinegar Relieves Headaches

People blame their headaches on many different organs of the body. Most headaches are blamed on the eyes, the nerves, the liver, the sinuses, the stomach, the bowel, kidneys or allergies and even the climate. Headaches can be put into two different classifications:

One type of chronic headache can be associated with toxic buildup and illness. A headache is an alarm telling the person that deep down in their body, destruction is going on. Pain and headaches are Mother Nature's great red flashing warning signal to take fast action! There may be trouble anywhere throughout the body. It could be in the liver, gallbladder, kidneys, bowel or any of the body's organs. It may be related to or caused by sensitive sinus, allergy, or alcohol problems, etc. See pages 54-58 to detox.

Avoid these headache trigger foods:

- *Additive and chemical-laced foods*
- *Salty, sugary or wheat-based foods*
- *Dairy foods, especially cheese*
- *Caffeine-containing foods*
- *Condiments, sulfites, MSG*
- *Alcohol, beer, wine*

– Linda Page, N.D., Ph.D., Author of *Healthy Healing*
See her informative website: *www.healthyhealing.com*

The **second type** of headache is emotional! This is often caused by nervousness, anxiety, stress, strain, tension or any personal or emotional upsets. This is a world where we must be associated with other human beings. Your daily life with others can throw you into many upsetting emotional problems because they can arouse emotions of fear, jealousy, envy, hate, greed, self-pity or self-indulgence. When emotions reach a boiling point, you can usually end up with a dull, throbbing headache. The worst headache is the migraine, which causes the sufferer to feel as if their head is splitting. **Do read these Bragg Books for more health guides:** • *Miracle of Fasting* • *Bragg Back Fitness* • *Build Nerve Force* • *The Bragg Healthy Lifestyle*. See back pages for booklist.

We have found in our many years of research on all kinds of headaches that when the body triggers a headache, the urine is alkaline rather than the normal acid. The kidneys are disturbed by the emotions and it means the body is off-balance. The fast working malic acid of ACV can help relieve headaches by aiding the kidneys to return urine to normal (average 6.4 pH) acidity.

Vaporized ACV can also help relieve headaches. In a vaporizer or small pan, put 2 Tbsps. ACV and 2 cups purified water. Bring mixture to a boil. As vapor begins to rise, turn heat off, put towel over head and lean over steam, taking 5 deep slow breaths of ACV steam vapors. Also try hot & cold vinegar compresses to forehead & entire neck area, then do some shoulder/neck rolls and massage head and shoulders, and if needed visit your Chiropractor. For pain use Bromelain 500 mg (available health stores) – it acts like aspirin without the toxic stomach upset. Many chronic headache sufferers have told us they get blessed relief with this method. By doing these things and faithfully following The Bragg Healthy Lifestyle, you will have no need for commercial headache remedies and pain killers!

Wise Health Advise from Dean Ornish, M.D. www.ornish.com

We tend to think of advances in medicine as being a new drug, a new surgical technique, a new laser, something high-tech and expensive. We often have a hard time believing that the simple choices that we make each day in our diet and lifestyle can make such a powerful difference in the quality and quantity of our lives, but they most often do. My health program consists of four main components: exercise, nutrition, stress management, love and intimacy and these four promote not only living longer, but living better.

Apple Cider Vinegar for Feet – Combating Corns, Callouses and Warts

For Corns and Callouses: First soak affected areas in warm water with $1/3$ cup ACV for 20 minutes. After soak, rub areas briskly with coarse towel, then gently use a pumice stone or wand. Now apply full-strength ACV- soaked gauze bandage overnight, and in the morning prepare a fresh ACV soaked bandage for daytime use. These treatments help soften and dissolve corns and callouses. Check shoes for comfort and fit. Wrong shoes are main cause of corns, callouses, bunions and blisters. For casual wear, Birkenstock shoes are great and use orthotic inserts when needed. Give yourself weekly pedicures, massages and exercise feet daily. Doing this while watching TV is ideal. Treat yourself to foot reflexology therapy (page 92). Walking barefoot on sand, grass and at home is beneficial. Be good to your feet – they carry you through life! We kept the famous foot doctor going strong and alert to almost 100 years young!

Dr. Scholl thanked us for our health teachings and said: "*The Bragg Foot and Health Books* are the best!"

For Common Warts: Use the ACV treatment, but caution: *do not rub warts, as this could spread them!* After soaking, use ACV-soaked gauze, cover with waterproof tape, keep on overnight. In the morning, for daytime treatment, apply a castor oil-soaked gauze bandage. At night you can alternate ACV with vitamin E (prick open capsule). Combination treatments work wonders readers write! If warts still become a problem, some doctors freeze them with liquid nitrogen. This method is fast, safe, easy and usually leaves no scars.

Apple Cider Vinegar Zaps Sore Throat & Laryngitis

Organic, raw ACV is a dangerous enemy to all kinds of germs that attack the throat and mouth! To fight the germs and keep the throat healthy, an ACV gargle mixture works miracles (1 tsp. to $1/2$ glass water). Gargle 3 mouthfuls of mixture each hour, then spit it out. Don't swallow the gargled mixture, because ACV acts like a sponge, drawing out throat and mouth germs and toxins.

As the throat feels better, gargle every 3 hours. We have famous singers, rock and roll bands to Metropolitan Opera's dynamic Jerome Hines, eternally youthful Beach Boys, Bette Midler and the popular Katy Perry using ACV to keep their throats healthy and germ-free. It's important for singers, teachers, ministers, public speakers and you!

Along with the gargling, we use an ACV wet compress as follows: first, place a thin ACV-soaked cloth over throat area, cover with Saran Wrap, then use a flat hot water bag or moist, hot wrung-out towel to heat the area, allowing ACV to absorb through the skin. This ACV hot compress is also great for cleansing and healing chest area when treating all lung congestions: colds, flu, bronchitis, emphysema, chest pains and asthma. It feels good, too.

Even in good health, use ACV gargle twice weekly to remove any body toxins being eliminated through the throat tissues. The gargle is also helpful during fasting, when the throat may produce a stringy mucus as part of the detoxifying process! Read our *Miracle of Fasting* book: it contains the powerful health message of fasting to detox, cleanse and renew the body. See pages 54 to 58.

Apple Cider Vinegar for Healthy Skin

Reap vitality with the apple cider vinegar massage: To a small basin of warm distilled water, add $1/2$ cup of ACV. Dip both hands in mixture and massage this all over your body (in shower or bathtub): face, neck, chest, arms, shoulders, back, abdomen, legs and feet. Massage mixture into skin thoroughly, be gentle on the face. This leaves skin soft and pH balanced. Healthy skin has an acid reaction, for it's throwing off toxic poisons through its billions of pores. (Skin is often called your third kidney.) After thoroughly wetting the skin with the mixture several times, rub and massage until the skin is dry. Do this at least twice a week and do not wash it off; leave it on the body. As you massage the mixture into the skin, you will feel a new vitality coming into your body.

Also soaking in an ACV bath restores the acid to alkaline balance in your body. If baths are not your thing, try mixing one cup of ACV and warm water in a spray bottle and spray yourself after a shower, rub it in and feel refreshed!

The reason this treatment is far better than using soap is because soap has an alkaline reaction on the skin and you don't want that! By keeping the skin in an acid reaction, it will help you have healthier skin. I've never used soap on my face or body, just ACV and it's worked wonders. If you use soap – use health soaps only.

We find after hard exercise or long mental work that we get a new feeling of strength and energy after one of these ACV massages. Also try gentle dry skin brushing with loofah pad or vegetable brush next time you feel mentally or physically tired (pg. 92). It helps remove old skin cells and toxic wastes. We know you'll want to do it often. The health benefits of improved circulation are obvious!

ACV Cleanser & Toner for Skin Problems

To open the pores and loosen dirt and grease from your face, turn off heat under a pan of steaming ACV water (3 Tbsp. ACV to quart purified water). Steam face over pan and use towel draped over head to trap steam. Then pat ACV on face with cotton ball to remove the loosened dirt. Repeat steaming and cleansing twice. Then you can gently squeeze out any blackheads. Then pat or spray on chilled ACV, diluted with equal amount of distilled water (store ACV mixture in refrigerator) to close pores and tone skin. Do steam cleansing twice weekly, as needed. Another excellent cleanser and toner is aloe gel or try fresh aloe vera cactus pulp. Cut off 1 inch of aloe vera rib, slit open and rub yellowish pulp directly on the skin. We grow our own aloe plants – you can grow them in pots also. Aloe is a great healer for burns, pimples, sores, bites, etc!

Apple Cider Vinegar for Sunburns

Gently pat undiluted ACV on skin to give relief from sunburn. Leave it on to help prevent blistering and peeling. For all-over sunburns, pour 1 cup of ACV in cool bath water, then enjoy the healing soak. After soaking, gently dry body, then pat ACV directly to needed areas. Wait 5 minutes, then pat on aloe vera gel. We receive many wonderful ACV testimonials *(pages a-d, 11, 23, 25, 29, 35, 37-38, 111-117 & visit web: bragg.com).*

We must always improve, renew, rejuvenate ourselves; otherwise, we harden. – Johann W. Goethe

Younger Looking Skin in Minutes With Apple Cider Vinegar Skin Tonic & Facial

The skin consists of microscopically small, flat scales that constantly flake off, thereby revealing the new skin beneath the outer, older layer of scales. In millions of people, the old, tired, dead, dry outer scales do not peel off promptly, slowing new growth and leaving their skin dry, sallow, dull and lifeless. This is known as "the old-age look".

Men and women can use this ACV skin tonic facial on their face and skin (50% ACV and 50% distilled water) weekly for amazing results! First, wash skin in warm water (no soap). Next, apply a wrung-out, hot water-soaked cloth to the face for 3 minutes, then remove. Soak thin cotton wash cloth in warm ACV water (1 Tbsp. ACV per cup of water) and again apply to face. Cover ACV-soaked cloth with cotton towel wrung out in hot water. Now lie down for 10 minutes or longer with your feet elevated up on the couch, against the wall, or use a slant board or an ironing board. This brings more blood circulation to revitalize the face for cell rejuvenation.

Remove both cloths and gently rub skin upwards with a coarse towel or our favorite – a small loofah face pad. This rub removes the hundreds of old, dry skin scales that have been detached and loosened by the ACV facial. You can repeat this weekly or as needed. Your skin will look as youthful as Cleopatra and will shine like a polished apple with new life. We should all have pride in looking our best and presenting a good personal appearance. You will be truly amazed and proud of yourself with the results from these age-reversing, simple health treatments!

I've been using Bragg Organic Vinegar and Bragg Organic Olive Oil for 10 years instead of expensive skin products. I'm 53 and my skin and face are soft and so youthful looking, people often ask me what I do. I tell them about Bragg's Vinegar and Olive Oil for their skin and body. Thank you so much. – Pat Williams, Ingelwood, CA

Sad Facts: Many people go throughout life committing partial suicide – destroying their health, skin, heart, youth, beauty, talents, energies and creative qualities. Indeed, to learn how to be good to oneself is often more difficult than to learn how to be good to others. – Paul C. Bragg

Skin Problems and ACV Treatments

ACV can be used to effectively relieve the pain and discomfort of **cold sores and genital sores** caused by the herpes virus. Apply ACV directly to the affected areas and the itching and burning discomfort will rapidly dissipate. ACV also helps the sores to heal more quickly.

Shingles and chicken pox, caused by herpes zoster virus, can be relieved with straight ACV compresses, also helps **psoriasis**. Gently apply to itching and burning areas. A cup of ACV in a warm bath also helps soothe itching.

ACV relieves the itching and discomfort caused by **poison ivy and poison oak** and other poisonous plants. Mix equal parts of ACV and distilled water and spray on affected areas to stop pain, itching and ease the redness and swelling. Keep ACV spray mixture in refrigerator; a cold spray is more soothing. (Read bottom of page 25.)

Healing is faster for **minor cuts and abrasions**, and there is less chance of infection if you swab areas daily with ACV (perfect disinfectant & healer, pg. 32). ACV also helps stop bleeding by helping the blood to clot. Soak a cotton ball in ACV and press on abrasion until bleeding stops.

Varicose veins can be unsightly and painful, but applications of ACV help shrink veins, and also take Vitamin C, K and Rutin. Wrap an ACV-dampened cloth around needed areas morning and night, then elevate legs, leaving on 15 minutes (follow instructions page 23). Then remove wrap, legs still up – start at ankles to gently press over pooled veins to get blood back into circulation. To help speed up inner cleansing and healing, remember to drink and enjoy your delicious Bragg Apple Cider Vinegar cocktail 3 times daily (page 96).

Relief from **dry, itchy skin and hives** will come after applying a paste of ACV and cornstarch to affected areas. The ACV paste mixture draws out the itching as it dries.

Oily skin can be helped by the ACV drink and the facial treatment twice a week, explained on page 22.

To help prevent **windburn, sunburn and chapping** coat the exposed skin with a mixture of 50/50 ACV and Bragg Organic Olive Oil mixture. When in the weather elements, carry this mixture along in a small bottle.

ACV for Insect Stings, Bites, Ear Infections, Acne, Psoriasis, Virus, Yeast & Fungus Problems

ACV helps stop pain and itching from **mosquito bites, insect bites, bee stings, head lice** and **jellyfish stings** and neutralizes their venom. Use straight ACV on affected areas or diluted ACV compress as needed. ACV helps **middle ear infections** and **swimmer's ear**, a condition from swimming and showering, which may cause temporary hearing loss. Dilute ACV with equal parts distilled water and drop into ear for **ear infections**, **earaches** or if you feel an **ear blockage**. This solution also treats chronic inflammation of the eardrum. Drug stores stock ear dropper syringes. If ear and skin problems persist, it is best to see a health professional.

For **hemorrhoids and rectal itching**, soak cotton ball in ACV or witch hazel and gently press area for relief.

Yeast and fungus infections of the body and mucus membranes (such as thrush in the mouth and throat, and the genital areas of males and females – especially children – such as **diaper rash** and **jock itch; athlete's foot, acne, psoriasis and eczema**) can all be treated with a 50/50 solution of ACV and distilled water. For athlete's foot, soak feet in 50/50 mixture of ACV and lukewarm water twice daily; for mouth thrush, gargle every 3 hours with 1 tsp. ACV in half glass of warm water. Also slowly drink a warm Bragg ACV cocktail morning and night. For genital areas, especially in the case of itch or diaper rash* on infants, swab affected area carefully with a solution of 1 Tbsps. ACV to 1 quart warm distilled water 3 times daily. The treatments for all yeast infections should continue for at least 10 days or until symptoms dissipate.

I have suffered from Psoriasis and Acne for 10 years. Since I started the ACV drink my skin looks better than ever. My rough spots are clearing and new skin is growing to replace the older patches. I am a Bragg fan for sure!!! – Cathrine Westergaard, NY

I have suffered with toe nail fungus for years, to the point the nail separates from the toe. For the last 10 months I have been soaking my feet for 15 minutes each night in your vinegar. The results are astounding. My nails are growing back smooth and clean of fungus. It sure works. Thank you. – Bill White, Corpus Christi, TX

*****ACV *helps heal rashes on humans – babies, children, adults, even animals. Also try aloe vera, witch hazel, calendula, comfrey and MSM ointments.*

Japanese Researchers have found that Apple Cider Vinegar inhibits the growth of the nasty E.coli bacteria.

Apple Cider Vinegar for Dandruff, Baldness, Itching Scalp, Dry and Thinning Hair

The high acidity (organic malic acid) plus the powerful enzymes (the "mother's" life chemicals) in ACV kill the bottle bacillus, a germ responsible for many scalp and hair conditions. The problems caused by this are dandruff, itching scalp, thinning hair and often baldness.

Every hair has its own oil can. Bottle bacilli can clog these tiny openings. Scales and small dry crusts are formed, resulting in itching and dandruff. The oil-starved hairs either fall out or break off, causing hair thinning and baldness. ACV not only kills bottle bacillus, but stimulates the oil cans for healthier activity. **For dandruff:** put 2-3 Tbsps. ACV in cup – part hair in sections and sponge ACV directly on scalp and wrap head with towel. ACV helps restore proper acid/alkaline balance to scalp, do before every shampoo. **For dry hair:** weekly apply castor oil or Bragg Olive Oil to hair, and ACV to scalp, then wrap. Leave on for 30 minutes to 3 hours before shampooing. **Hair growth stimulating mixtures:** for bald and thinning areas try these 2 mixtures: • On scalp (2 Tbsps ACV and tiny pinch cayenne powder), apply hour before shampooing (keep out of eyes!). • Mix royal jelly cap, tiny pinch cayenne & 1 tsp ACV & pat on bald areas – leave on overnight. Many get great results.

Hair rinse mixture: for a healthy after-shampoo rinse for shine and body, add $1/3$ cup ACV to quart of water. Pre-mix in handy plastic bottle and keep in shower to use.

For Muscle Soreness and Aching Joints

To soothe tired, aching muscles and joints, there is nothing like an ACV bath combined with a self-massage. While soaking in a warm bath with 1 cup ACV added, massage entire body, starting at feet. Gently squeeze and relax each part of the foot, working slowly up right leg to hip, then left leg. Continue up torso, arms and neck, always rubbing toward the heart. For the face, lightly stroke skin in upward direction; avoid pulling facial skin down. Finish with firm fingertip dry massage in circular motions over the scalp, then finger rub your entire ears.

For pain & stiffness, arthritis, osteoarthritis & to help heal & regenerate cartilage & bones use glucosamine & chondroitin sulfates & MSM combo, works miracles!

For Arrhythmia and Heart Strengthening

The heart, a large muscle and your master pump uses large amounts of potassium to keep going strong for your entire life! It's the hardest working muscle in the body (bottom page 6). It must have a constant, continuous supply of power and energy to continue beating. ACV contains a natural chemical that combines with heart fuel to make the heart muscle stronger and helps normalize blood pressure and cholesterol. Recent studies show ACV helps remove dangerous artery plaque! To help arrhythmia also take Magnesium Orotate and the heart combo of CoQ10, Folic Acid, B6 and B12. Also enjoy your basic 3 ACV cocktails daily. (See page 96 for details).

Low Fat Meals Cut Heart Disease Risk

A great British research report by Dr. George Miller of Britain's Medical Research Council stated: *"High fat meals make the blood more prone to clot within 6 to 7 hours after eating. Low fat meals can almost immediately reverse this condition. Most heart attacks occur in the early morning. One reason may be the overnight clotting effects of a high fat dinner. Researchers feel by cutting fats from diet, you may be able to add years to your life and cut risk of heart disease!"* University of Chicago and Stanford's research supports Miller's statement that the healthy heart, plant based low-fat vegetarian meals with ample fresh fruits, salads and vegetables are the best and safest! (See Healthy Heart Habits page 87.)

How to Improve the Digestion

Millions suffer indigestion (gerds), which is aggravated by poor digestion and weak saliva juices. This causes distress: gas, heartburn, burping and stomach bloating. Before mealtime, sip $1/3$ tsp. Bragg ACV. Hold in mouth for a minute before swallowing. This promotes enzymes and saliva, which improves the digestion that starts in the mouth. This causes stomach digestive fluids to flow faster, resulting in improved digestion and better health. ACV also protects against food borne pathogens.

Bragg Organic Apple Cider Vinegar with the "mother" is vital to the body's digestive balance by stimulating the flow of precious enzymes and saliva in the mouth. I recommend to stop heartburn, gerds, gas indigestion and also improve digestion, sip $1/3$ tsp. Bragg ACV before meals to activate flow of digestive juices. – Gabriel Cousens, M.D., *Author, Conscious Eating*

Chewing Gum Habit Causes Stomach Problems

Please never chew gum because it fools the body into thinking food is coming. Chewing starts precious digestive juices flowing. These powerful juices can cause trouble with your empty stomach's lining, resulting in ulcers, stomach problems, heartburn, bloating, gas, etc.

Fight Kidney and Bladder Problems

Avoid all animal, dairy, salt, coffee, alcohol and sugar products. All ages should follow The Bragg Healthy Lifestyle for health. Use ACV on salads and have your ACV drink 3 times daily. ACV can help bladder problems and dissolve some types of stones. Drink 8 glasses of distilled water, plus some organic, unsweetened cranberry juice. Add $1/3$ tsp. ACV to each glass, which helps acidify urine, inhibits bacterial growth and promotes healing. You may sweeten the cranberry drink with organic grape juice, raw honey or Stevia. You can also do 2-3 day watermelon only flush. Thoroughly chew or grind the seeds, too. This is a great kidney and bladder cleanser and healer!

28

For bedwetting: Mix $1/2$ to 1 tsp. buckwheat honey with $1/2$ tsp. ACV before bedtime. It's also best to stop liquids 3 hours before bedtime, except for small sips.

For all kidney and bladder problems: Children and adults should drink 8 glasses daily of distilled water. It's important for urinary tract and kidneys. Have ACV drink (page 96) and this healing drink: 2 Tbsp fresh or dried corn silk to 1 quart distilled water or try marshmallow herbal tea, 2 to 3 times daily. Add $1/2$ tsp. ACV to each cup and sweeten with 1 tsp. buckwheat honey. (Save dry corn silks from fresh corn & store in airtight bottle.)

To soothe and heal bladder infections: Add 1 cup ACV to warm low sitz bath. Use 1 to 2 times daily. Also, ACV douches help (page 30). Use a Dipstick self-tester from drugstore to check if you have a urinary track infection. *****

To eliminate "dribbles": To keep the bladder and sphincter muscles tightened and toned – urinate – stop – urinate – stop, 6 times, twice daily when voiding. This simple exercise works. After age 40, do this every day.

**Important: We don't endorse antibiotics, but if you ever take them, please take acidophilus liquid or capsules to replace the friendly bacteria in your body.*

Apple Cider Vinegar Combats Gallstones

Before starting the 2 day gallbladder flush, prepare for 1 week by drinking slowly – upon arising, at mid-morning, mid-afternoon and after dinner – $1/2$ tsp ACV with a 6 ounce glass of apple juice; or if hypoglycemic or diabetic, then dilute with half distilled water. Organic, unfiltered apple juice is rich in malic acid, potassium, pectins and enzymes. These act as solvents to soften and help remove debris (small stones, etc.) and cleanse the body. Doctors have non-surgical methods for removing the difficult, larger stones using sound waves. But it's best to purge small and medium-sized ones twice yearly as they can grow to cause problems! (see testimonies page 114)

During the 2-day gallbladder flush no food is eaten, only liquids. Combine in 8 oz glass: $1/3$ Bragg Organic Olive Oil (no substitutes), $2/3$ apple juice (organic) and 1 tsp. Bragg Organic ACV. Drink this mixture 3 times the first day. *At night, sleep on your right side when on flush, pulling right knee toward chest to open pathway.* On the second day, take mixture twice. On both days drink all the organic apple juice desired, but no water or any other liquid. (*This gallbladder flush is not for diabetics unless supervised by a health professional.*)

About midmorning on the third day, eat a raw variety salad (nature's broom) of cabbage, carrots, celery, beets, tomatoes, sprouts and lettuce, with lots of ACV and olive oil. If desired, have bowl of lightly steamed greens, kale, collards, chard or any leafy greens. Season with Bragg ACV, Bragg Olive Oil, nutritional yeast flakes and spray of Bragg Aminos – this gives delicious flavor to greens.

We take this miracle cleanser flush at least once or twice a year. Check your bowel movements for tiny, greenish-brown stones. This flush will amaze you what your gallbladder, stomach and colon will clean out!

29

Your book "Apple Cider Vinegar" saved me from having my gallbladder out. The specialist wanted to take my gallbladder out, instead I followed your apple cider vinegar flush and it worked along with healing prayers at church! I think all book and health stores should carry your vinegar book. I am grateful for you writing it. God bless you. – Carmen Puro, Traverse City, MI

Distilled water plays vital part in treatment of illness, arthritis, etc. – Dr. Banik

When on flush nausea may occur. This shows toxins, mucus and bile are being dumped in the stomach. Your body wants it out! If nauseated, your body is saying: "Drink 1 to 2 glasses of purified water and regurgitate until your stomach is empty." (You might have to depress your tongue while leaning over the bowl.) Once it's out, you will feel better right away! Remember, it's always wisest decision when nauseated to get out whatever is causing an upset stomach, whether at home or even in a restaurant restroom!

Apple Cider Vinegar Helps Shrink Prostate

With a fork, "whip" 2 Tbsps. ACV with 2 Tbsps. Bragg Organic Olive Oil, a dash of Bragg Liquid Aminos and cinnamon. Use this ACV mixture daily over salads, sliced tomatoes, avocados and steamed veggies. Enjoy with meals, zinc-rich raw pumpkin seeds. Also take Zinc, Prostex and Saw Palmetto supplements which are healers for the prostate.

Apple Cider Vinegar for Female Troubles

For healthier vagina, use ACV healing douches and baths when needed. ACV pH acidity is same as vagina's. ***Douche mixture:*** 3 Tbsps. ACV to 2 quarts warm purified water is a cleansing, healing douche. If discharge, yeast infection or vaginitis is present, use 1-2 times daily as needed. ***For bath:*** Add 2 cups ACV to water. ***Sitz Bath:*** Add 1 cup. ***Hotflashes, PMS, UTI:*** drink ACV 3-5 times daily (pgs. 96, 111). ***To shrink, tighten and tone flabby womb muscle:*** Eat raw garden salads (pg. 97). Sprinkle Bragg Organic ACV, Bragg Organic Olive Oil, and Bragg Sprinkle (24 herbs & spices), then spray Bragg Aminos over salad. Daily do kegel and Bragg Posture Exercises (page 79), walks, yoga, etc.

"PAP" Vinegar Tests Pinpoints Cancer

Vinegar can help identify cervical cancer in women says Johns Hopkins University along with 15 other studies. A vinegar swab test instead of a Pap Smear, gives fast results (cancer area goes white) and costs only a fraction making it affordable, especially in developing countries.

Fight Arthritis with Apple Cider Vinegar

Hard, stony deposits fill up, cement, enlarge and cripple the joints! Crippling, painful arthritis and joint problems are the sad result! Flush out those stony crystals with your daily ACV drinks. Upon arising, an hour before lunch, and dinner have delicious ACV cocktail (pg. 96) as follows:

30

Stir 8 ounces distilled water with 1 to 2 tsps. equally of ACV and raw honey (diabetics use Stevia). Also add ACV to your salads and steamed greens. Be faithful to The Bragg Healthy Lifestyle and your 24 hour fasts. Eat 60% to 70% healthy, raw foods (organic is best), drink 8 glasses daily of distilled water (free of chemicals and inorganic mineral). To help heal and regenerate, take natural multi-vitamin-minerals, Braggzyme (page 124-125), Glucosamine, Chondroitin and MSM supplements, plus alfalfa tablets and 1 to 2 tsps. cod liver oil daily. Improvements are amazing, plus enjoy 2 organic apples daily to keep the doctor away!

Apple Cider Vinegar Combats Mucus

Millions have postnasal drip and are plagued with toxic mucus in their sinus cavities, nose and throat, which is most uncomfortable! If mucus sufferers remove all dairy products, eggs and sugars from their diet, follow The Bragg Healthy Lifestyle, take a weekly 24-hour fast and use ample ACV, soon these mucus conditions will vanish on this healthy toxicless and mucusless diet!

Upon arising, have glass of warm distilled water with 1-2 tsps. ACV and 1-2 tsps. raw honey (recipe page 96). Also enjoy this drink midmorning and mid-afternoon. On your salads use 1 to 2 tsps. ACV combined with Bragg Olive Oil and a dash or spray of Bragg Liquid Aminos. Try our delicious, all-purpose Bragg Aminos in the handy, small spray bottle. This is a great method for seasoning salads, potatoes, vegetables, etc., and even popcorn! The spray bottle is perfect to take along when dining out!

For throat gargle and nasal wash: Add 1 tsp. ACV to glass warm water for throat gargle (pg. 20) or nasal sniff wash to help clean out mucus. Sniff or use dropper up right nostril, roll head back, then side to side, lean over, blow out mucus. Then repeat with other side. Do 3x daily until mucus conditions subside. Along with the ACV drink, enjoy fresh carrot and green juices between meals. It's important to sip and savor fresh juices slowly, as they are really foods, not just beverages. Small amounts of juice (or food) in the mouth at one time will be better digested and more easily used by the body chemistry.

ACV mouthwash: 1 tsp ACV to glass of water kills mouth bacteria, fights plaque and tartar. Promotes healing, freshens breath and helps prevent gum disease (bottom pg. 38).

Vinegar Bandages Stop Bleeding & Infection

Studies show vinegar soaked bandages quickly stop bleeding and prevent infection. The Army is currently testing these new bandages where urgency is so important to save lives. Dad and I have had many miracle healings with vinegar for burns, cuts, bites, etc. as thousands of our readers have.

For Nosebleeds: Soak cotton ball or gauze in ACV and lightly pack in nostrils. Relax, sit down and lean forward for 10 min. (breathe through mouth) pressing nostrils together while ACV pack helps blood congeal. Repeat if needed. Vitamins C, K and Rutin are helpful. Be sure to drink 8-10 glasses of pure water daily – nosebleeds are often caused by dehydration.

Apple Cider Vinegar and Constipation

It's important that the bowels move regularly and freely! Outgo should equal intake. You should have a bowel movement soon after arising and within an hour after meals. Flaxseeds and its' tea with ACV act as bowel lubricants, as do fresh fruits, prunes, vegetables and distilled water.

Make the ACV-Flaxseed Bowel Lubricant Mixture: Boil two cups distilled water with 4 Tbsps. flaxseeds for 15 minutes or soak overnight. Mixture becomes jellylike when cold. Stir 2 Tbsps. of mixture, plus 1 tsp. ACV in 8 oz. distilled (hot or cold) water (add maple syrup or honey if desired sweetened). Drink upon arising and hour before bed. Store mixture in refrigerator and use when needed.

For Healthy Elimination: Use miracle Psyllium Husk Powder. Add 1 Tbsp. of this cleansing herb to any of these: Bragg ACV drink, juice, distilled water, herb tea, soups, etc.; let it soak 2 minutes before drinking or eating! This helps cleanse mucus along small intestine and colon walls and pulls toxins from intestinal tract. Also use Bragg Organic Olive Oil over salads, veggies, potatoes, etc.– it helps elimination and detoxifies the colon, plus adds delicious flavor to foods.

To Check Bowel Elimination Time: Have some fresh or frozen whole corn with your evening meal. Purposely don't chew all the kernels. (Always chew food thoroughly otherwise.) Check stools to see when corn is eliminated, usually within 14 hours. When it's cleansed of toxins and malnutrition is treated, the body becomes healthier and more normal. Because constipation brings on serious health problems, including arthritis, it's important to keep the pipes (colon and arteries) clean and open by faithfully following Bragg Healthy Lifestyle.

For easier-flowing, healthful bowel movements:

It's natural to squat to have bowel movements. It opens up the anal area more directly. When on toilet, putting feet up 6 to 8 inches on waste basket or footstool gives the same squatting effect. Now raise and stretch your hands above your head so that the transverse colon can empty completely with ease. It's important to drink 8-10 glasses of pure water daily! (Read page 87 and take your psyllium husk powder daily.)

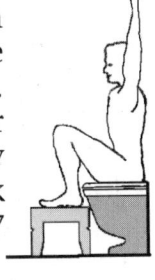

The body is 70% water and pure, steam-distilled (chemical-free) water is important for total health. You should drink at least 8-10 glasses of water daily. Read *Water – The Shocking Truth That Can Save Your Life*, for more info on importance of purified/distilled water. See back pages 120-121, 127 for Bragg Health Booklists.

What Becomes of the Acid Crystals Precipitated in the Body That Age Us?

You have often heard the expression, "He's stiff and old and his flesh is tough." When you think of "old" people you usually think of them as having stiffness in their body, with tough, brittle flesh (see Dr. Carrel's study on page 10). Why do people get stiff in the joints and their flesh tough when they have added birthdays to their life? Most people would answer this complex question with the remark, "Because they are old". But this isn't the real answer why people get stiff joints and tough flesh. The answer to premature ageing is unhealthy living and potassium deficiency! People rarely study their bodies or learn what to eat for healthy tissues and youthful joints (ACV brings miracles). They are satisfied to eat what agrees with them. Or they eat foods they were reared on as children and carry these early eating habits (sadly often unhealthy) right into their adult life and then into their children's lives!

WATER IS KEY TO HEALTH & ALL BODY FUNCTIONS:

• Elimination	• Muscles	• Nerves
• Circulation	• Metabolism	• Energy
• Digestion	• Assimilation	• Sex
• Bones & Joints	• Heart	• Glands

Rearing Healthy Children is Important

The Bragg family children, grandchildren and great-grandchildren have all been reared on The Bragg Healthy Lifestyle. We were taught to keep in perfect health so that the body tissues would remain soft and tender and have elasticity and health. This correct way of eating enables us to come to the later years of life with youthful looking skin, keen hearing, sharp, sparkling eyes and perfect mental, emotional and physical health, for a long, useful, healthy, and fulfilled happy life.

Miracles with Apple Cider Vinegar

The members of the Bragg family follow The Bragg Healthy Lifestyle. They have learned the lessons of good nutrition and the miracles of ACV for themselves and their animals. The children were impressed when Farmer Bragg would have an old hen prepared for dinner. The old hen's meat was tough and didn't taste good. This is what happens to poultry and beef when it is deficient in potassium. Human flesh suffers the same problems.

To prove to the children conclusively that apple cider vinegar and honey needed to be an important part of their daily nutrition, he would then select another old hen for the dinner table. This time he fed that old hen ACV faithfully twice a day, for ten days. When the hen was prepared for the dinner table, the children tasted the difference in the old hen's meat. They noticed how tender it was – just like a young hen and they asked for second helpings. *(P.S. Most of the Bragg family members are now happy, thriving, heart-healthy vegetarians!)*

Animals and pets can greatly benefit from the use of ACV: from cats and dogs to parrots, chickens, horses and even cows. It deters insects such as fleas, tics and mosquitoes; relieves skin and ear problems; prevents intestinal upsets; reduces excess weight; promotes a healthy shiny coat; eliminates cat urine odor and even can take away the smell of stinky skunks!

Children are very responsive to healthy lifestyle changes, and those start with providing the right foods (fruits, vegetables, whole grains and reasonable amounts of other healthful snacks), encouraging regular exercise and activity and limiting television, video and web watching!
– Susan K. Rhodes, Ph.D., Medical University of South Carolina

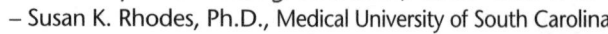

"Apple Cider Vinegar Cures Burns"

A testimonial from **Joel** & **N'omi Orr**, Chesapeake, VA: We have used Bragg's Apple Cider Vinegar for several years and love your wonderful book about it. We want to share with you something that we believe is one of the greatest benefits Bragg's Organic Apple Cider Vinegar brings to humanity *(commercial vinegars don't have the same effect)*: Bragg's Apple Cider Vinegar, if splashed on a burn of any kind, stops the intense, continual pain instantly and permanently! It also prevents scarring & infection! We not only keep a bottle in our kitchen, we also keep bottles in our cars to use when people get burned from hot engines, radiators, etc. When traveling, we have helped burn victims from accidents in restaurant kitchens, cars, etc. We suggest everyone keep a bottle of your vinegar nearby! Everyone who has tried it, has praised it. Bragg's Vinegar is the best burn healer in the world, no matter how bad the burn! We thank you! The Joel Orrs, Chesapeake, VA

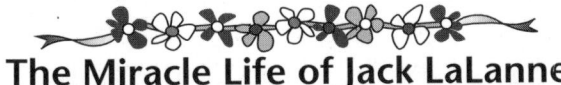

The Miracle Life of Jack LaLanne

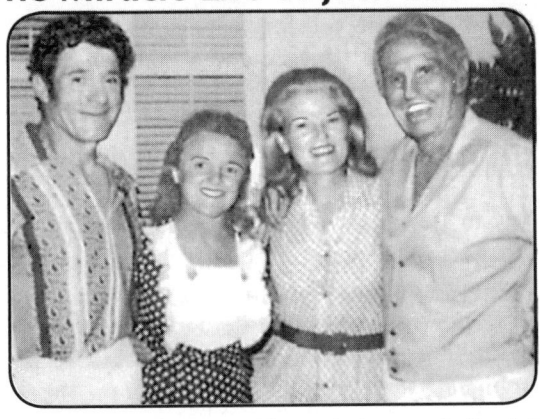

Jack LaLanne, Patricia Bragg, Elaine LaLanne & Paul C. Bragg

Jack says he would have been dead by 16 if he hadn't attended The Bragg Crusade. Jack says, *Bragg saved my life at age 15, when I attended the Bragg Health and Fitness Crusade in Oakland, California.* From that day, Jack has continued to live The Bragg Healthy Lifestyle, inspiring millions to health, fitness and a long and happy life! *See web: www.jacklalanne.com*

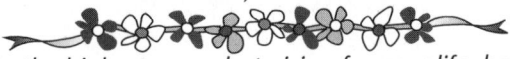

Create the highest, grandest vision for your life, because you become what you believe. – Oprah Winfrey

All Through Life You Fight Acid Crystals

When acid crystals harden in the joints and tissues, the joints become stiff and the tissues hardened. Also meat becomes tough and tasteless. When the animals are given apple cider vinegar regularly, the precipitated acid crystals enter into a solution and pass out of the body, thus making the body tissues healthier and tender. This applies to human flesh also. Now, when body tissues hold all the precipitated acid crystals they can, the crystals then appear in the bursae and the joints of the body, resulting in bursitis and arthritis. 1 to 2 tsps. apple cider vinegar with 1 to 2 tsps. raw honey in glass of distilled water 3 times daily (pg.96), will help relieve stiff, aching, prematurely old joints. You be the judge. See how elastic and flexible all your joints become!

Keep Your Joints and Tissues Youthful

Most people have lost their normal contact with Mother Nature and simple, natural living. They no longer know how to eat the simple way God intended. If you suffer from prematurely old joints and hardened tissues, be sure to take the ACV mixture three times daily. Eliminate or cut down on animal proteins. Stop all refined sugars, products and beverages! Soon you will see how youthful your body and joints begin to feel.

Toxic Acid Arthritic Crystals Make Joints Grind

The grinding sound you hear in your neck when you roll your head is the toxic arthritic acid crystals that have deposited themselves on the uppermost bone of your spine – the Atlas. Just as ACV washes sludge off windows, it also washes the body sludge from the joints and cardiovascular system of the body. Fasting, and taking the Bragg's Apple Cider Vinegar Cocktail (page 96) will help eliminate acid crystals from the joints. A feeling of agelessness gradually will replace that tight, stiff, ageing feeling. You will start to feel more flexible, pain-free and loose in every moveable joint of your body.

Loving thoughts are little seeds . . . Let them blossom into deeds.

Roses are God's autograph of beauty, fragrance and love. – Paul Bragg

ACV Helps Banish Stiffness From Body

You will find, after several months of the ACV and honey cocktail taken 3 times daily – that the stiffness and misery will be gone from your joints and body. You will discover you can walk or run up several flights of stairs without any effort and pain. Also follow page 87. You will notice that you look, act and feel younger!

Make The Bragg Healthy Lifestyle a life-long daily habit! Over the years we have seen many stiff-jointed, prematurely old people transform themselves into new, youthful, healthy people! We can't do it for you. You must make the effort to give this ACV and Bragg Healthy Lifestyle a chance to prove what it can do for you!

Questions About Apple Cider Vinegar

Many people have some preconceived idea that apple cider vinegar is harmful to the body. Instead it's the distilled, pasteurized, filtered, the malt and synthetic, dead vinegars that must be avoided for human consumption!

Let us assure you that there is nothing in this wonderful, organic, raw ACV that can in any way harm your body! People ask us about the merits and benefits of ACV. See the inside front cover for a list of some of the miracles it can perform and has for centuries.

Animal proteins and fats have a tendency to thicken the blood, while the natural acids and enzymes in ACV help to keep the blood healthier and thinner. Also, that's why people naturally crave and serve cranberry sauce, which contains four different natural acids, with turkey and other fowl. They serve applesauce with roast pork dishes and a slice of lemon with fish, or steak with mushrooms, all rich in natural acids, like Apple Cider Vinegar.

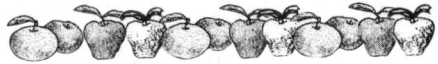

Bragg Organic Apple Cider Vinegar is the #1 food I recommend for maintaining the body's vital acid-alkaline balance and healthy digestion.
– Gabriel Cousens M.D., Author of *Conscious Eating*

I started using Bragg's Organic Apple Cider Vinegar and have never felt better. My joint pain and stiffness is fast disappearing and my energy level has improved. I am sold on it for life. Thank You! – Joseph M. Cole, Illinois

ACV Helps Normalize Blood Pressure

Natural food acids served along with animal proteins are designed to lessen the blood thickening influence of these heavy proteins. In order for blood to circulate freely throughout the body, it must be thin. When blood thickens, it strains the heart. The blood pressure then goes up and a host of other health problems begin.

Remember, blood has to circulate all over the body through the arteries, blood vessels and tiny capillaries. It's impossible for blood to circulate freely through these hair-like pipes when it is thickened with too many heavy protein meals, fats, hardened oils, etc.

Several years ago, we met a woman with extremely high blood pressure. We put her on a two day ACV, honey and water fast program with nothing to eat for 48 hours. She had an ACV cocktail 5 times daily, plus 5 glasses of pure distilled water – total of 10 glasses. In 48 hours, her blood pressure had dropped to almost normal! The buzzing in her ears ceased, and her dull headache stopped. After a short period of correct eating (no salt, sugar, saturated fats, tea, coffee, etc.) combined with Bragg Healthy Lifestyle, Fasting and ACV Program, her blood pressure was normal and she felt reborn!

People also ask us if ACV will make them slender. It helps balance body chemistry and normalizes body weight. We have been using the ACV program in the Bragg family for over five generations and it has brought wonderful results for our health and our trim bodies!

I started taking Bragg ACV and within days I noticed my blood pressure unbelievably lowered. I told all my friends in my community and bought a bottle of Braggs ACV for close friends. – Dr. Qasim Hussain Shah, Malaysia

Evidence reveals ACV has shown to lower blood pressure & strengthen the heart muscle because it acts as a blood thinner, plaque remover & reduces risk of strokes & heart attacks. It also contains important potassium & enzymes which are vital & needed to keep the heart & bloodstream healthy.

WORLD'S #1 MEMORY MAN THANKS BRAGG ORGANIC VINEGAR
that gives him an amazing, healthy brain and miracle memory abilities! He says Bragg Apple Cider Vinegar cleans the dendrites and brain cables and keeps his brain healthy. He shares this message with students world-wide.

Studies show low CoQ10 levels cause heart disease, declining memory and brain function and gum and periodontal conditions.
– Dr. Stephen Sinatra, Coenzyme Q10 Phenomenon www.sinatramd.com

The Bragg Healthy Lifestyle Promotes Super Health

The Bragg Healthy Lifestyle consists of eating 60%-70% fresh, organic, live foods: raw vegetables, salads, sprouts, fresh fruits and fresh juices; raw seeds and nuts; 100% whole grain breads, pastas, cereals, nutritious beans and legumes. These are the good (no cholesterol, no fat, no salt, no sugar) "live foods" – the body fuel required for lively, healthy people! This is the reason people become revitalized and reborn into a fresh, new life filled with joy, health, vitality, youthfulness and longevity! There are millions of Bragg Healthy Lifestyle followers around the world! When it works for you, please write and share your results with us, we love hearing from our book friends!

Five Generations of Healthy Braggs Give Thanks to Using Apple Cider Vinegar

Since birth, all the Bragg children have used ACV. They fed it to their children and now their grandchildren are feeding it to the great-grandchildren! We all use ACV along with Bragg Organic Olive Oil on our salads. We put both on our steamed greens (cabbage, chard, collards, kale, spinach, mustard and beet greens, broccoli, Brussels sprouts and cauliflower) and use with many other foods.

Millions of our students around the world have used ACV and never once has anyone reported a negative reaction from using it. In fact, they sing its praises! So, you also will soon see the benefits from using Bragg ACV and following The Bragg Healthy Lifestyle Program.

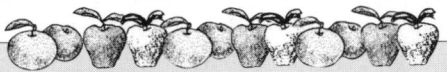

"All vinegar is not created equal. Bragg Organic Apple Cider Vinegar is made from fresh, crushed organic apples and then matured in wooden barrels. It's smoother and so much healthier than other vinegars. Apple cider vinegar is healthful because it's loaded with vitamins, minerals and rich in potassium. Apple Cider Vinegar helps balance the body's vital acid/alkaline balance.
. . . Do As I Do – Drink Bragg's Apple Vinegar Drink 3 times daily! "
– Julian Whitaker, M.D., Health and Healing Newsletter • www.drwhitaker.com

The universally accepted #1 fruit, the apple, is popular across America and around the world. Early American settlers, the Pilgrims, brought apples to America in the 1600s and became Johnny Appleseeders, starting apple orchards that eventually spread throughout America.

Apple Cider Vinegar and Arthritis

People ask if ACV cures arthritis. This is not possible, for curing is an internal biological function that only the body can perform. We have seen miracles how ACV fights arthritis. A healthy diet, with ACV, exercise, deep breathing, rest, relaxation and living The Bragg Healthy Lifestyle are required to put the body in a condition to cure itself. ACV is an important part of this program (page 30). When all Mother Nature's supreme forces are used, the body will turn from sickness to wellness. Super health is something you must desire, seek out, earn and always guard and treasure it for your life's health sake!

Apple Cider Vinegar Relieves Muscle Cramps

Many people are awakened in the middle of the night with sharp, painful muscle cramps. These often occur in the feet and lower or upper legs. Sometimes they occur in the stomach, intestines and occasionally in the heart. These are frightening experiences! Most people who experience leg cramps are forced to jump out of bed and pound or firmly massage the area to get relief. Many people with cramps in other parts of the body have to walk quickly to get relief. When precipitated acid crystals get into the circulation of the legs and other parts of the body, they can cause severe cramps. We recommend taking 2 tsps. ACV and 1-2 tsps. raw honey (page 96) in glass of distilled water three times daily to relieve these painful cramps. This allows the precipitated acid crystals to enter into a solution and pass out of the body, causing cramps to cease. Calcium and also magnesium orotate supplements taken before bedtime can also help prevent cramping, plus they help promote a sounder sleep.

Acid Crystals Cause Premature Ageing

Everyone, even the healthiest person in the world, must continually fight the buildup of acid crystals in the body. The strongest enemy of acid crystals is the organic apple cider vinegar, raw honey and distilled water cocktail. This powerful mixture puts the acid crystals in solution so they can be flushed out of the body by the kidneys and other organs of elimination.

Take This 48 Hour Test

For 2 full days, take nothing into your system but liquids. Have the ACV cocktail 3 to 5 times daily, plus another 4 to 5 glasses of distilled water daily as well. Ample water is needed to flush the toxins out!

On the second and third day, after you have eaten nothing else for 48 hours, take a sample of your first morning urine and store in labeled bottles with tight lids. Keep on shelf for 2 weeks, then examine sediment at bottom of bottles. These are some of the disease-causing toxins that were flushed out of your body!

Potassium – The Master Mineral

Always keep in mind the fact that potassium puts toxic poisons in solution so they can be flushed out of the body. **The body is self-cleansing, self-correcting, self-repairing and self-healing!** Just give it the tools to work with and soon you can enjoy a painless, tireless, ageless body, regardless of age! Forget age and calendar years, for age isn't toxic! You age prematurely when you suffer from malnutrition and potassium deficiencies. These cause low Vital Force and waste buildups and poor elimination that causes disease to proliferate.

The Bragg Healthy Lifestyle will help you rebuild your Vital Force. Watch the transformation that will take place in your body when you faithfully follow your ACV regimen. You can and will create the kind of person you want to be! Plan, plot and follow through! Start now!

Although you must follow this program closely, please don't try to do everything listed immediately. Remember, it took you a long time of living by wrong habits to cause any of the problems your body might have now. So, it's going to take time for the body to cleanse, repair and rebuild itself into a more *perfect healthy home* for you! Please remember, your body is your temple while on this earth, so cherish it and protect it!

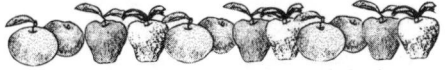

Many studies show people who lower their blood cholesterol levels by diet can slow, or even reverse atherosclerosis and cut the risk of having a heart attack.
– University of California, Berkeley Wellness Letter • www.berkleywellness.com

WE THANK THEE

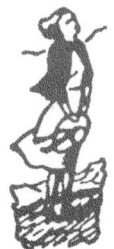

For flowers that bloom about our feet;
  For song of bird and hum of bee;
For all things fair we hear or see,
  Father in heaven we thank Thee!
For blue of stream and blue of sky;
  For pleasant shade of branches high;
For fragrant air and cooling breeze;
  For beauty of the blooming trees;
Father in heaven we thank Thee!
  For mother love and father care,
For brothers strong and sisters fair;
  For love at home and here each day;
For guidance lest we go astray,
  Father in heaven we thank Thee!
For this new morning with its light;
  For rest and shelter of the night;
For health and food, for love and friends;
  For every thing His goodness sends,
Father in heaven we thank Thee!
  – Ralph Waldo Emerson

42

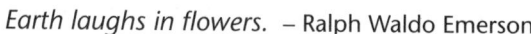

Earth laughs in flowers. – Ralph Waldo Emerson

*A strong body and a bright, happy or serene countenance can
only result from the fine admittance of thoughts of joy and
goodwill and serenity into the mind.* – James Allen

Where there is no vision, the people perish. – Proverbs 29:18

*Fasting is an effective and safe method of detoxifying the body –
a technique that wise men have used for centuries to heal the sick.
Fast regularly and help the body heal itself and stay well!*
– James Balch, M.D., Co-Author *Prescription for Nutritional Healing*
"Bragg Books were my conversion to the healthy way."

*It never hurts to brush up on the three Rs:
Respect for yourself. Respect towards others.
Responsible living today, tomorrow and always!*

If you love Nature, you will find Beauty everywhere. – Vincent Van Gogh

*A book is a garden, an orchard, a storehouse, a party, a mentor,
a teacher, a guidepost, a counsellor.* – Henry Ward Beecher

My father and I have shared The Bragg Healthy Lifestyle Blueprint with millions of people around the world at the Bragg Health and Fitness Crusades. I would now like to share it with you as part of the Apple Cider Vinegar Health System.

With Blessings of Health, Peace, Joy and Love,

Patricia Bragg

The Bragg Healthy Lifestyle
The Bragg Blueprint for Physical, Mental and Spiritual Improvement – Healthy, Vital Living to 120.
– Genesis 6:3

by
Patricia Bragg, N.D., Ph.D.
Life Extension Educator & Pioneer Health Crusader

Just think, in only 90 days you can build a new bloodstream! Not a thick, sluggish, toxin-saturated bloodstream, but a rich, red bloodstream, healthy in all the vitamins, minerals and vital nutrients necessary for radiant and long lasting health. First and foremost, we must build the health content of our bloodstream. This is one of the great secrets of life: The more healthy nutrients in your bloodstream, the more oxygen is going to flood into your body, purifying its cells. Oxygen is the greatest natural stimulant. It stimulates, but doesn't depress. Unnatural stimulants stimulate, but there is an aftermath of depression! Tobacco, alcohol, coffee, tea, refined white sugar and flour and drugs (prescribed, street and over counter) have this bad effect on the body, but not God's oxygen – it's the invisible health staff of life!

So, in The Bragg Healthy Lifestyle we forever discard these harmful, destructive stimulants. You are going to be strong and never allow these to enter your body again! You are going to rely on the many wonderful, natural stimulants to create a more healthy vital force.

Man's days shall be to 120 years. – Genesis 6:3

First, you are now going to start breathing deeper and slower, as it's important for super energy! Then you are going to eat organic, live foods, such as fresh salads, fruits and vegetables and freshly squeezed juices, that will build up your blood health and energy.

Before you eat or drink anything, I want you to ask yourself this important question, "Is this going to build a healthy bloodstream or destroy it?" Be on the alert to protect your precious river of life - your bloodstream! When it demands liquids, give it the best – pure distilled water or live-food juices, such as fresh organic fruit and vegetable juices. Get yourself a juicer. Every day fortify your blood with fresh orange, grapefruit and fruit or carrot and green juices or combine juices such as celery, tomato, beet and parsley or see page 65. Three of the best juices to add to vegetable juices are raw spinach, cabbage and watercress. For a taste delight, add juice of 1 – 2 garlic buds (wrap in veg leaf to juice), excellent purifier and heart protector.

Do not consume too much of these powerful, live-food juices. One to two pints a day is more than enough! Some people get a juicer and overdo it. Overloading your body with juices can upset your delicate blood-sugar balance. Eating the whole fruit is still the best! Just because something is good for you doesn't mean that a lot of it is. As with all things in life, moderation of your food intake is best for building Vitality Supreme!

Imagine: In just a short 11 months you will have an absolutely New You! The billions of soft cells that make up eyes, nose, skin, hands and feet, as well as all the vital organs of your body, will be renewed. You do not need to submit to the huge risk of heart, kidney or any other dangerous transplant operations!

You have within your power, through the food you eat, the liquid you drink and the air you breathe, the ability to build a fresh, vital body from the top of your head to the tip of your toes. What you eat and drink today will be walking and talking tomorrow! How wonderful our Creator has been to us, to give us the miracle power every 90 days to build a new bloodstream and every 11 months, an entirely new body!

It's Never Too Late to Seek and Build Radiant Health!

The Creator gave us the intelligence and reasoning power to take control of our body! But the flesh is dumb! You can stuff anything in your stomach and almost get away with it until the day of reckoning arrives! Most young people live this way, because they believe they are totally indestructible! But what a sad lesson they learn after 40 or 50 years of wrong living! The infirmities and the aches and pains creep into their bodies, making life miserable and proving to them that their dream of indestructibility was a myth and a lie!

Live by the reasoning mind, rather than by the senses of the body. The dumb senses are constantly enticing you to do the very things that destroy your wonderful body. Look around you at the sad, broken-down human sights you see. Weak people, mentally depressed people and sickness everywhere! The average person's suffering – it's sad but true – is self-inflicted . . . a slow, self-murder!

Whatsoever a man soweth, he shall also reap. – **The Bible**

We should know and observe the fact that everything in the universe is always governed by definite laws. If we understand and follow these universal laws we will sow the seeds of constructive, healthy living!

Make every day a healthy day and each day you will improve! You will feel new strength and energy flooding into your body. The feelings you will experience when you live 100% The Bragg Healthy Lifestyle are indescribable! What an incredibly powerful and joyful feeling it is to be fully alive and vigorous, with unlimited energy and powerful nerve force. An amazing example is ageless Jack LaLanne who is filled with energy! (pg. 35)

Weak people find weak excuses to continue living their unhealthy lifestyle. They will tell you they are too old to begin The Bragg Healthy Lifestyle Program. Age has no force, nor is it toxic! Time is just a measure. Long ago, the Bragg family gave up living by calendar years. We only live by biological years and we feel ageless!

Millions Suffer from Premature Ageing

There are millions in their 30s and 40s who are, sad to say, prematurely old biologically. Yet there are many people in their 70s, 80s and 90s who are biologically youthful, active, healthy and happy! *The second half of life is best!*

In our opinion, if you are experiencing premature ageing, you are suffering from a highly toxic condition and you are suffering from unnecessary nutritional deficiencies. These are the main causes of most human troubles. The Bragg Healthy Lifestyle will show you how to banish these vicious enemies. From this minute on, stop living by calendar years! Just forget your birthdays, as we do. All of us are reborn every second of the day as new body cells are being constantly created.

Cease this talk of getting old! From this minute on, you will have no age except your biological age and this you are going to control. Every day say to yourself . . .

I Will Stay Youthful, Active, Happy and Healthy!

46

Say it repeatedly, burn it deeply into your mind and it will sparkle all your days for your entire long happy life!

Most people have a dreadful fear of getting old. They picture themselves half blind, hearing impaired, with teeth gone, energy and vitality spent or senile. They see themselves as a burden to their family and friends. They envision themselves in the nursing home alone, forgotten, with Alzheimer's disease.

Despite the fear of old age and the train of ailments that go with it, you can prevent this human tragedy. You can skip this terrible period by changing how you live from this day forward! Today is the day to prepare against becoming senile and decrepit. That is why I urge you to follow the wise and wonderful laws of Mother Nature. You will grow younger as you live longer! That is what this health program is all about: The preservation of your precious vital health for a long, fulfilled life!

Every man is the builder of a temple called his body . . . We are all sculptors and painters and our material is our own flesh and blood and bones. Any nobleness begins at once to refine a man's features, and any meanness or sensuality to imbrute them. – Henry David Thoreau

Wise Prevention Helps Keep You Healthy, Youthful and Vigorous!

Lengthening life by special treatment for chronic miseries often means merely adding years of ill health and misery to a person's life. This is often called *the living death*. Who wants to extend life just to suffer? We say, the healer's function is to prevent sickness and disease. No person is able to heal you! Only you can heal yourself! In order to be healthy it's essential to learn how to live healthy in order to be healthy always. They say –

An ounce of prevention is worth a ton of cure!

My father and I always stress to our readers that prevention is always the healthiest, the best and is priceless!

Diet for health and youthfulness – Your diet should be composed of 60% to 70% raw fruit and raw or steamed, baked or wokked vegetables. By this habit, such conditions as stomach upsets, miseries and constipation, which occur often in children and adults, can be avoided (pages 32-33). Output should equal intake. You should have a bowel movement soon upon arising and after each meal.

The greatest enemy of health is constipation, but this can be eliminated by a diet that gives you sufficient bulk, moisture, lubrication and vigorous exercise of the entire abdominal cavity (pages 33, 73). In remote parts of the world, where we traveled beyond influences of so-called modern civilization, mankind indulges in the normal habit of defecation after every meal. I want you to train yourself to have a bowel movement soon after arising and after each meal. Children can be taught this important healthy habit from infancy. Living The Bragg Healthy Lifestyle faithfully, constipation vanishes!

The Body is The Hero

"It is the body that is the hero, not science, not antibiotics. . . not machines, drugs or new devices. . .The task of the physician today is what it has always been, to help the body do what it has learned so well to do on it's own during its unending struggle for survival to heal itself!
It is the body, not medicine, that is the hero!
– Ronald J. Glasser, M.D., Author, *"The Body Is The Hero"* (amazon.com)

The natural healing force within us is the greatest force in getting well.
– Hippocrates, Father of Medicine, 400 B.C.

Constipation is Your Health's Worse Enemy

Studies reveal the presence of toxic poisons in cases of constipation. When these toxins are absorbed into the general circulation, the liver "your detoxifying organ" is unable to cope with them. These toxins are then thrown back into the body to cause degenerative diseases, toxemia, cancer, premature ageing, sickness and lack of energy, etc.

Your lifestyle and diet play a vital role in maintenance of health, good elimination and the prevention of disease. Research shows that diets composed of refined white flour and sugar; preserved meats, as hot dogs and luncheon meats; white rice; coffee, tea, cola drinks and alcohol; margarine; overcooked vegetables; high fat, sugared, salted, and processed foods create serious health problems, especially in the colon and intestinal tract, heart and respiratory areas. It's wise to never eat refined, processed, embalmed and dead, unhealthy foods!!!

Your Energy is Your Body's Spark Plug

48

Your energy comes from the spark of life, which is maintained by the atomic energy contained within every single cell of the human body. It embodies electrons, protons and neutrons. They are constantly discharging their ionic compounds as energy is expended in work or play, whether mental or physical, in accordance with natural laws. This energy loss must be replaced. Every cell in your body is like a battery that, when run down, must be recharged. Primarily, this is done through the intake of food, proper breathing, rest and exercise which helps recharge your billions of cells.

Now, there are two kinds of food: The first is in a low rate of health vibration, like the fast junk foods we mentioned: the processed, chemicalized, dead foods, as in refined white flour and sugars, etc. It's impossible to have a youthful, dynamic body when, year after year, you feed it food and drinks with a low rate of vibration.

Perfect health is above gold; a sound body before riches. – Solomon

In nature there are neither rewards or punishments – there are consequences!

Pray for wisdom in your daily living, for more faith and for more patience with yourself and others before you pray for just things.

The Bragg Healthy Lifestyle Program consists only of **foods** in a **high rate of health vibration.** Many have the preconceived idea that animal protein is the highest rate of food. While protein is an important nutrient to the body, healthier vegetarian protein is best. Organic fresh fruits and vegetables have high health vibrations. Fruit produces blood sugar, which helps to feed the nerves of the body. Fruit has a two fold purpose in the body. First, it's rich in blood sugar; second, it's an important detoxifier and destroyer of harmful toxins that can do the body harm.

Allergies are Often The Body Cleansing

Often you will hear people say, "I am allergic to apples, grapefruit, peaches, strawberries, etc." These people have no idea what these foods are doing in their bodies. To give you an example, when my father Paul C. Bragg was reared in the South, his typical diet was rich in animal proteins and fats from hogs, chickens, cows and sheep they raised. At each meal, they had a variety of these meat proteins. I'm sad to say that accompanying these dishes were white flour biscuits, bread, fried potatoes and inevitably, a heavy, sugary dessert.

When he attended this military school (page 14) from age 12 on, his body became so saturated with toxic poisons, mucus and putrid food residues that, when he ate fresh fruits, he suffered not only hives, but also colds, headaches and pains as well. These were erroneously thought to be allergic reactions! But were natural self-cleansing responses of his body that wanted him healthy and clean! The cleansing fruits were pushing out the mucus and toxins through his skin, lungs, etc.! He avoided eating these vital foods until he became a health advocate at age 16. Only after he had been cleansed and purified with healthy foods, apple cider vinegar and faithful fasting one day a week, and occasional longer fasts – it was then he could enjoy fresh fruits and vegetables without negative reactions.

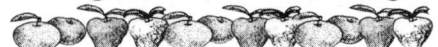

There is much false economy: those who are too poor to have the seasonable fruits and vegetables, will yet have pie and pickles all the year. They cannot afford apples, yet can afford tea and coffee daily. – Health Calendar, 1910

One physician told medical students to be leery of all new drug research. – Sandra Tanenbaum, Professor of Hospital & Health Services, Ohio State University

Through fasting and careful nutrition, he slowly detoxified himself and could eat all the wonderful, natural foods without experiencing the allergic cleansing reactions of his youth. His early TB was the outcome of these wrong foods. For this reason, people who have been living on a diet high in animal proteins, fats, salt, starches and refined sugars can't immediately include a large amount of fresh fruits and vegetables in their diet. It's best to slowly ease into The Bragg Healthy Lifestyle to allow the body to cleanse itself gently.

Health Transition Diet – Everyone who wants to live the healthy life must thoroughly understand just what is going on in their body chemistry. Fresh, organic, raw fruits and vegetables help flush the toxins out. The body can't be rushed. It takes the average person a long time to saturate the body with toxic poisons. Now it's going to take time to flush this debris out with this transition diet!

The more organic raw fruits and raw vegetables that you condition yourself to handle, the more cleansed your body will become! So, recognize these foods, which are in the highest rate of healthy vibration. But please, also respect their cleansing and detoxifying action!

> **We often eat 100% raw meals of fruits, vegetables or salads for a few days, but usually our meals are 60% to 70% raw:**

Breakfast: Fresh, raw juice (orange, grapefruit, or carrot, celery, garlic, spinach, etc.) or raw fruit (in season, melon, apricot, berry, peach, nectarine, etc.) or the nutritious, delicious Bragg Energy Smoothie, on page 96.

Lunch: Large variety salad with fresh greens, vegetables, sprouts and a few raw nuts or seeds (sunflower, sesame, pumpkin, almonds, pecans, walnuts, etc.). See page 97.

Dinner: Variety salad, followed by two steamed, baked or wokked fresh vegetables and one of the following: beans, lentils, brown rice, whole grain pasta, tofu (soybean curd), baked or steamed potatoes.

Remember to get your daily ACV into your diet with the ACV Cocktail and sprinkle ACV over steamed greens, cauliflower, squash, broccoli, cabbage, stringbeans, etc. It is also especially delicious on garden variety salads.

People are told they must start the day with a big breakfast, to give them great energy in the morning hours. So, they gorge themselves on processed cereal with milk and sugar; ham and eggs; or bacon and eggs; stacks of hot cakes or buttered toast and jelly. All of this is washed down with coffee, milk or cocoa. You will note that there are no fresh fruits at this meal.

Only a person doing the most strenuous physical labor could possibly burn up a meal like this, and I doubt that even they would. All the vital energy of the body will be needed to digest these heavy animal proteins and fats, refined starch and white sugar breakfasts. All too often, they lie in the stomach like a ton of bricks and have to be dynamited out. Now you know why there is so much indigestion and constipation and why laxatives are one of the biggest sellers in drugstores!

How can a big meal like this give a person strength for their morning duties? The truth is, it can't! This is how parents and, consequently, their children are brainwashed by the big food interests who sell all their commercial, sugared, unhealthy, worthless foods. You must change your ideas about food! Learn to eat in moderation. It's important you not overfuel your body. If you overfeed your body, you clog it up. A diet of healthy, organic, raw foods with a high rate of vibration will help keep your insides clean and you healthier!

51

Vegetarians are Healthier and Live Longer

Most uninformed nutritionists call meat the #1 source of protein. Those proteins coming from the vegetable kingdom are referred to as the #2 proteins. This is a sad and terrible mistake! It should be the other way around! In this day and age, almost all meat is laden with herbicides, fungicides, pesticides and other chemicals that are sprayed on or poured into the feed which these animals consume. They are also pumped full of hormones, antibiotics, growth stimulators and toxic drugs to fatten them up and keep them from dying from the unhealthy conditions they live in! Beware of all animal products!

In regions where meat is scarce, cardiovascular disease is unknown. – Time Mag.

Fast Foods, processed meats and sugared foods up weight and medical bills!

Bragg Veg. Cookbook has over 700 healthy delicious recipes – see pgs.119 & 121.

Eliminating Meat is Safer and Healthier

Play it safe, become a healthy vegetarian. Look what they feed cattle – the dead, ground up carcasses of other feed lot animals who, for a variety of reasons, didn't make it to the slaughterhouse.

Speaking of the slaughterhouse scene, what kind of chemical reaction do you suppose would occur in your body if somebody put a choke chain around your neck to keep you in line, shoved you onto a conveyor belt, and made you watch in horror as all of those in line in front of you were beheaded one by one? Well, your body would be pumped so full of adrenaline from all that fear you wouldn't know what hit you! Unused adrenaline is extremely toxic. If you think for a minute that most of the meat that you consume is not packed with this toxic substance, you are sadly mistaken!

Also, consider the fact that cattle, sheep, chickens, etc., are all vegetarians. When you eat them, you are just eating polluted vegetables. Why not skip all the waste and toxins and just eat healthy, organic vegetables?

And what about that myth that you have to eat meat to get your protein? If that were true, where do you suppose farm animals, especially horses, get their protein? They are vegetarians! They get their protein from the grains and grasses that they eat. You are no different. You can get the proteins you need from the large variety of whole grains, tofu, raw nuts, seeds, beans, fruits and vegetables that God put on this planet for your health. Study the Vegetable Protein % Chart, (Page 53).

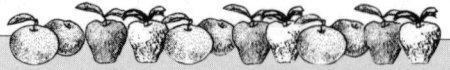

A truly great book teaches me better than to just read it. I must soon lay it down and commence living its wisdom. What I began by reading, I must finish by acting!
– Henry David Thoreau

Whatsoever was the father of disease, an ill diet was the mother. – Herbert, 1859

Millions of Americans are committing slow suicide with their unhealthy, inactive lifestyle; heavy meat eating, high sugar and fat diets; plus smoking, drinking alcohol and doing drugs – all this damages their organs and the inside of their arteries, adding graver health problems to their lives! – Patricia Bragg

Vegetarian Protein % Chart

LEGUMES	%
Soybean Sprouts	54
Soybean Curd (tofu)	43
Soy flour	35
Soybeans	35
Broad Beans	32
Lentils	29
Split Peas	28
Kidney Beans	26
Navy Beans	26
Lima Beans	26
Garbanzo Beans	23

VEGETABLES	%
Spirulina (Plant Algae)	60
Spinach	49
New Zealand Spinach	47
Watercress	46
Kale	45
Broccoli	45
Brussels Sprouts	44
Turnip Greens	43
Collards	43
Cauliflower	40
Mustard Greens	39
Mushrooms	38
Chinese Cabbage	34
Parsley	34
Lettuce	34
Green Peas	30
Zucchini	28
Green Beans	26
Cucumbers	24
Dandelion Greens	24
Green Pepper	22
Artichokes	22
Cabbage	22
Celery	21
Eggplant	21
Tomatoes	18
Onions	16
Beets	15
Pumpkin	12
Potatoes	11
Yams	8
Sweet Potatoes	6

GRAINS	%
Wheat Germ	31
Rye	20
Wheat, hard red	17
Wild rice	16
Buckwheat	15
Oatmeal	15
Millet	12
Barley	11
Brown Rice	8

FRUITS	%
Lemons	16
Honeydew Melon	10
Cantaloupe	9
Strawberry	8
Orange	8
Blackberry	8
Cherry	8
Apricot	8
Grape	8
Watermelon	8
Tangerine	7
Papaya	6
Peach	6
Pear	5
Banana	5
Grapefruit	5
Pineapple	3
Apple	1

NUTS AND SEEDS	%
Pumpkin Seeds	21
Sunflower Seeds	17
Walnuts, black	13
Sesame Seeds	13
Almonds	12
Cashews	12
Macademias	9

Data obtained from *Nutritive Value of American Foods* in Common Units, *USDA Agriculture Handbook No. 456.* Reprinted with author's permission, from *Diet for a New America* by John Robbins (Walpole, NH: Stillpoint Publishing)

The Miracle of Fasting
Master Key to Internal Purification

If you do a complete water fast for 24 hours each week, soon you will be able to add more fresh fruit and vegetables to your diet. After a fast of 3 or more days, then you can include more foods that are in a high rate of vibration.

I faithfully fast for 24 hours every Monday and the first three days of each month. Wait until you experience this! You will greatly benefit from the inner cleansing and will love the pure, clean, healthy feeling you receive!

Fasting Cleanses, Renews and Rejuvenates

Our bodies have a natural self-cleansing and healing system for maintaining a healthy body and our "river of life" – our bloodstream. It's essential that we keep our entire bodily machinery from head to toes in perfect health and in good working order to maintain life! Fasting is the best detoxifying method. It's also the most effective and safest way to increase elimination of waste buildups and enhance the body's miraculous self-healing and self-repairing process that keeps you healthy.

If you prepare for a fast by eating a cleansing diet for 1 to 2 days, this can greatly help the cleansing process. Fresh salads, fresh vegetables, fruits and their juices, as well as green drinks (alfalfa, barley, chlorophyll, chlorella, spirulina, wheatgrass, etc.) stimulate waste elimination (page 96-97). Fresh foods and juices can literally pick up dead matter from your body and flush it out of the body!

Daily, even on most days during our fasts, our friend Linus Pauling inspired us to take 3,000 mg. of mixed vitamin C powder (C concentrate, acerola, rosehips and bioflavonoids) in liquids. This is a potent antioxidant and flushes out deadly free radicals that produce harmful effects, cancer, etc. Vitamin C also promotes collagen production for new healthy tissues and is especially important if you are detoxifying from prescription drugs or alcohol overload.

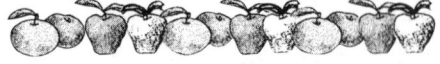

The body is self-cleansing, self-correcting and self-healing when you give it a chance with a fasting cleanse and living a healthy lifestyle!
– Patricia Bragg, N.D., Ph.D., Pioneer Health Crusader & Lifestyle Educator

Fasting Removes Sludge from Your Pipes

A moderate, well planned distilled water fast (our favorite) or a diluted fresh juice (35% distilled water) fast for beginners can also cleanse your body of excess mucus, old fecal matter, trapped cellular, non-food wastes and help remove inorganic mineral deposits and sludge from your pipes and joints. Remember your Vinegar drink also helps remove artery plaque. (See pages 63-66 for juice fasting and combination juices, etc.)

Fasting works by self-digestion. During a fast your body intuitively will decompose and burn only substances and tissues that are damaged, diseased or unneeded, such as abscesses, tumors, excess fat deposits, excess water and congestive wastes. Even a relatively short fast (1 to 3 days) will accelerate elimination from your liver, kidneys, lungs, bloodstream and skin. Sometimes you will experience dramatic changes (cleansing and healing crises) as accumulated wastes are expelled. With your first fasts you may temporarily have headaches, fatigue, body odor, bad breath, coated tongue, mouth sores and even diarrhea as your body is cleaning house. Please be patient with your miracle body! (See *bragg.com* – Bragg Fasting Book excerpts.)

After a fast your body will begin to self-cleanse and healthfully rebalance! When you follow The Bragg Healthy Lifestyle, your weekly 24 hour fast removes toxins on a regular basis, so they don't accumulate. Your energy levels will amazingly begin to rise – physically, psychologically and mentally. Your creativity will begin to expand. You will feel like a different person – which you are – for now you are being cleansed, purified and reborn. It's truly the Miracle of Fasting – read page 58!

Fasting Brings Miracle Longevity Results

Professor A. E. Crews Edinburgh University, who studied worms and animals, said: *"Given appropriate and essential conditions, including proper care of the body, Eternal Youth can be a reality in living forms! It's possible, by repeated processes of fasting, to keep an earthworm alive twenty times longer than normal and also proven with animals."* This proves the life-extending merits of fasting!

(See these important websites: www.walford.com and www.nobel prize.org/nobel_prizes/medicine/laureates/1912/carrel-bio.html)

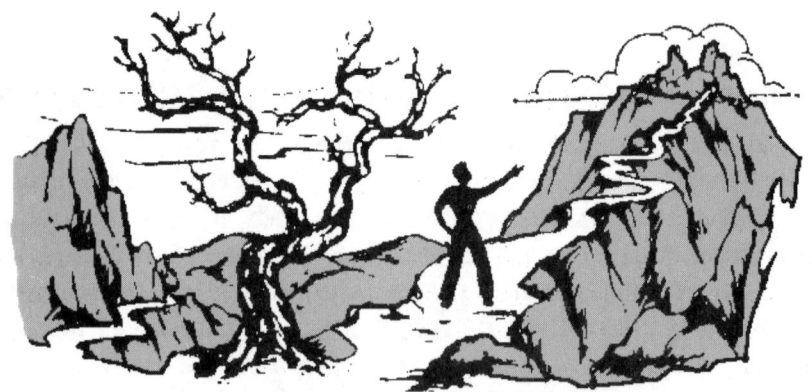

The Trail to Perfect Health

My father and I are very sincere about our fasting program. We know what it has done for us, for the members of our family, our friends, and millions of Bragg health conscious students all over the world. So The Bragg Healthy Lifestyle calls for 4 longer fasts a year, long with a faithful weekly 24 or 36 hour fast. I always fast the first 3 days of every month and all day each Monday. Also, I usually take my longer, cleansing fasts at the beginning of each season.

Remember, it took time for the body to build up toxins, so it takes time to cleanse and unload them! Take your time! Be faithful to The Bragg Healthy Lifestyle. You will reap wonderful, priceless, long-lasting health benefits. Please read our book the *Miracle of Fasting* as it gives many more details about the many benefits of fasting.

By relieving the body of the work of digesting foods, fasting allows the system to rid itself of toxins, while facilitating healing. Fasting regularly gives your organs a rest and helps reverse the ageing process for a longer and healthier life. (Bragg Books were my conversion to the healthy way.)
– James F. Balch, M.D., Co-Author, *Prescription for Nutritional Healing*

Eat Plenty of Raw Cabbage – Miracle Cleanser and Healer

Cabbage (raw) has amazing properties. It stimulates the immune system, kills bacteria and viruses, heals ulcers, and according to Dr. James Balch in Prescription for Cooking and Dietary Wellness, your chances of contracting colon cancer can be reduced by 60% by eating cabbage weekly. Dr. Saxon-Graham states that those who never consume cabbage were three times more likely to develop colon cancer. A Japanese study shows that people who ate cabbage had the lowest fatality rate from any cancer. Therapeutic benefits have also been attributed to cabbage in relation to scurvy, gout, rheumatism (arthritis), eye diseases, asthma, pyorrhea, and gangrene. See Bragg Raw Organic Vegetable Health Salad Recipe page 97. We love cabbage and also we make a variety of sandwiches wrapped in their leaves instead of bread. These cabbage wraps are so delicious!

Internal Cleanliness is the Secret of Health

What you want to strive for is a clean, toxicless body! Gradually include more organic fresh raw fruits and raw vegetables in your diet. Have fresh fruits in the morning and a large raw, combination vegetable salad at noon. If you like, you may have some fresh fruit for dessert. Eat a yellow vegetable, such as a yam, sweet potato, yellow squash or carrots, and a green vegetable every day. Cook vegetables by baking, steaming or wok (stir-fry) them. Remember to save some raw vegetables for your cleansing Bragg Raw Organic Vegetable Health Salad (on page 97).

With your main meal you may have and want a more concentrated form of protein. Our favorite and healthiest proteins are vegetarian! If you insist on eating animal proteins, have (hormone-free) not over 2 times a week. Your diet should include raw nuts and seeds: almonds, cashews, peanuts, pecans, pumpkins, sesame, sunflower, walnuts, etc. and avocados. Enjoy beans, brown rice and legumes, soybeans and tofu as often as desired. By having a variety of God's natural foods you will enjoy a balanced healthier diet and a long, healthier life!

57

You may use natural, cold or expeller pressed oils as: olive, flax, soy, safflower, sunflower and sesame. Read labels carefully before buying. I put Bragg organic extra virgin, cold pressed olive oil over my baked potatoes, instead of salt-free butter. It's also perfect over brown rice, lentils, beans and vegetables. Foods are extra delicious with a spray of Bragg Liquid Aminos, the perfect all-purpose health seasoning (contains 16 amino acids) – now available in spray bottles at health stores nationwide. Also, try Bragg Sprinkle and Kelp Seasoning and Nutritional Yeast (large flakes taste better), rich in B Complex and B12, page 124.

The best way to eat potatoes is baked. I use a fast method of baking. Thoroughly scrub potato (either white, yam or sweet). Don't wrap or oil it. Bake in a 450° oven for 25 minutes. This converts the starch of the potato to a blood sugar. Be sure to eat the skin, too! Baked this fast way, it's crunchy and delicious. I don't believe in microwaves that destroy food cells, as irradiation

---

The secret of longevity is eating intelligently. – Gaylord Hauser

BENEFITS FROM THE JOYS OF FASTING

Fasting renews your faith in yourself, your strength and Gods strength.
Fasting is easier than any diet. • Fasting is the quickest way to lose weight.
Fasting is adaptable to a busy life. • Fasting gives the body a physiological rest.
Fasting is used successfully in the treatment of many physical illnesses.
Fasting can yield weight losses of up to 10 pounds or more in the first week.
Fasting lowers & normalizes cholesterol, homocysteine & blood pressure levels.
Fasting improves dietary habits. • Fasting increases pleasure eating healthy foods.
Fasting is a calming experience, often relieving tension and insomnia.
Fasting frequently induces feelings of euphoria, a natural high.
Fasting is a miracle rejuvenator, slowing the ageing process.
Fasting is a natural stimulant to rejuvenate the growth hormone levels.
Fasting is an energizer, not a debilitator. • Fasting aids the elimination process.
Fasting often results in a more vigorous marital relationship.
Fasting can eliminate smoking, drug and drinking addictions.
Fasting is a regulator, educating the body to consume food only as needed.
Fasting saves time spent marketing, preparing and eating.
Fasting rids the body of toxins, giving it an internal shower & cleansing.
Fasting does not deprive the body of essential nutrients.
Fasting can be used to uncover the sources of food allergies.
Fasting is used effectively in schizophrenia treatment & other mental illnesses.
Fasting under proper supervision can be tolerated easily up to four weeks.
Fasting does not accumulate appetite; hunger pangs disappear in 1-2 days.
Fasting is routine for most of the animal kingdom.
Fasting has been a common practice since the beginning of man's existence.
Fasting is a rite in all religions; the Bible alone has 74 references to fasting.
Fasting under proper conditions is absolutely safe. • Fasting is a blessing.

58

Fasting As A Way Of Life – Allan Cott, M.D.
Fasting is not starving, it's nature's cure that God has given us. – Patricia Bragg

Spiritual Bible Reasons Why We Should Fast

Acts 13:2-3	Neh. 1:4	Luke 4:2-5, 14	Deut. 8:3-8	Matthew 9:9-15
Acts 14:23-25	Ezra 8:21	Luke 9:1-6, 11	Joel 2:12	Matthew 17:18-21
3 John 2	Gal. 5:16-26	Mark 2:16-20	Matthew 7:7-8	Deut. 11:7-14, 21
1 Cor 10:31	Gen. 6:3	Matthew 4:1-4	Psalms 119-18	Neh. 9:1, 20-21
1 Cor. 13:4-7	Isaiah 58:6, 8	Psalms 69:10	Psalms 35:13	Matthew 6:16-18

Dear Health Friend,

This gentle reminder explains the great benefits from *The Miracle of Fasting* that you will enjoy when starting on your weekly 24 hour Bragg Fasting Program for Super Health! It's a precious time of body-mind-soul cleansing and renewal.

On fast days I drink 8-10 glasses of distilled (our favorite) or purified water, (I add 1-2 tsps Bragg Organic Vinegar to 3 of them). If just starting, you may also try herbal teas or try diluted fresh juices with $^1/_3$ distilled water. Every day, even some fast days, add 1 Tbsp of psyllium husk powder to liquids once daily. It's an extra cleanser and helps normalize weight, cholesterol and blood pressure and helps promote healthy elimination. Fasting is the oldest, most effective healing method known to man. Fasting offers great, miraculous blessings from Mother Nature and our Creator. It begins the self-cleansing of the inner-body workings so we can promote our own self-healing.

My father and I wrote the book *The Miracle of Fasting* to share with you the health miracles it can perform in your life. It's all so worthwhile to do and it's an important part of The Bragg Healthy Lifestyle.

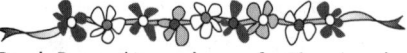 With Love, *Patricia*

Paul Bragg's work on fasting and water is one of the great contributions to The Healing Wisdom and The Natural Health Movement in the world today.
– Gabriel Cousens, M.D., Author of *Conscious Eating & Spiritual Nutrition*

also does. A fair priced, safer alternative is the convection oven. It's almost as fast as the deadly microwave and can be built in or placed on your kitchen countertop.

We never use table salt – it should have no place in your diet! Salt is an inorganic substance and only causes problems in the body! Organic sodium found naturally in "live" foods is best. Read labels and don't buy products that add salt!

Avoid Refined, Processed, Unhealthy Foods!

Eliminate refined, white flour products and white sugar products entirely. Eat no mushy, dead, refined cereals or those dry sugared cereals, etc. are unhealthy despite some being enriched with chemically produced vitamins and minerals. (Health Stores carry natural organic whole-grains cereals, granola, breads, rolls, pastas, even pastries.)

Avoid these foods: Fried, salted, refined, preserved and chemicalized foods; coffee, black and green (caffeine) teas, cola and alcohol drinks; sugared drinks, overcooked, oversalted vegetables and salted, creamed and white flour-thickened soups. Read page 86 for a complete foods-to-avoid list.

You now know the foods to avoid: Refined, unhealthy foods high in fat, salt and sugar; meat and dairy products; sugared foods and beverages and chemicalized water.

You now know the foods you can eat: Fresh fruits (organically grown is always best to buy or grow yourself); fresh juices; raw variety salads; fresh vegetables steam, bake or wok; vegetable proteins, beans, legumes, tofu, raw nuts, seeds, etc. If you really want animal and fish proteins, limit them to twice weekly. Occasionally, eat nothing but fresh fruits or fruits, raw vegetables and sprouts for 1 or 2 days a week. Remember, vegetarians are the healthiest among Americans! Research proves this! See web: *ornish.com*

Use your imagination to plan enjoyable, live food meals that are powerful for super health. Keep your meals simple! Avoid eating too many food mixtures. Don't overeat! Be moderate in all things for the best of health.

The men who kept alive the flame of wisdom, learning and piety in the Middle Ages were mainly healthy vegetarians. – Sir William Axon

Dr. Dean Ornish is able to reverse heart disease in over 70% of his patients who follow, among other things, a low-fat, healthier vegetarian diet. – ornish.com

Who is strong? He that can conquer his bad habits. – Ben Franklin

Eat only when you are really hungry, not because it is mealtime. Earn your food by activity, vigorous exercise and deep breathing. You will see how much more you really enjoy your food when you deserve and earn it!

The Miracle Powers of Fruits

Always keep in mind that the most perfect food for man is fresh, ripe fruits. Mother Nature, in her unique way, brings together in her fruits a marvelous balance. The fruits are living combinations of vital principles, in high rates of vibration, bio-magnetized, to release the living building blocks so necessary to maintain life.

Tinted by basking in the rays of the vitalizing sun, taking in draughts of magnetized air, drawing into itself vital minerals through its roots in the earth, delicious, organic fruits are God's perfect creations for man.

Man can duplicate the natural occurring chemicals of an apple in a chemist's dish, but he can't construct an apple! Man may analyze the minerals of a cherry, but he doesn't know what makes it red. He may take apart and try to reconstruct a grape, and find that the grape supports life, but the man-made chemicals do not!

Fruits contain bioelectric principles that give the electric sparks of life! Organic fruits are the most perfect foods from Mother Nature and God. Fruits will support life indefinitely to a superior degree when a body is cleansed and living in a natural environment. Ask your grocer to stock healthy organically grown produce.

Who has not had his mouth water when seeing a luscious dish of delicious, ripe fruit before him – for instance some yellow pears with a dash of pink or a beautiful bunch of tapering grapes, green, blue or red. The sight of fruits and the taste of them, more so, bring an abundant secretion of digestive juices, for fruits are the most natural foods. I can say without reserve that fruits are designed beautifully for our digestive tracts.

Organic fruits are filled with life for health, mind and body.

Every man is the builder of a temple called his body. We are all sculptors and painters, and our material is our own flesh and blood and bones. Any nobleness begins at once to refine a man's features, any meanness or sensuality to imbrute them. – Henry David Thoreau

I have seen a sick person turn down all other foods for some freshly squeezed orange juice. His sick body craved the nutrients in juicy oranges. I have seen children torn with fever ask for fruit juice. Why didn't they ask for a hot dog? Mother Nature's guidance was in force!

But diets that consist solely of fruits are impractical for the average American, although they would be splendid for short periods in a tropical climate. While we have come so far from our natural state that we can't maintain an efficient lifestyle as 100% fruitarians, we still need to eat plenty of fresh fruits! One of the many reasons I love Hawaii are the luscious tropical fruits! Plan a Hawaiian vacation soon and enjoy the free Bragg Exercise Class at Waikiki Beach in Honolulu. It's going strong, thousands of Bragg followers from around the world annually visit the exercise class, see info page iii.

I especially recommend ripe organic bananas, which are not a fattening fruit - as many thought. They are 70% water and are high in potassium. Organic apples of all kinds make excellent eating, as do pears, oranges and grapes. In the fall, winter and spring, eat organically grown dates, sun-dried figs, raisins, apricots, etc. along with fresh fruits. When you eat fruits, see how light and wonderful you feel and look and your energy zooms!

Avocado is Mother Nature's Miracle Food

The avocado tree is strong and insects don't bother it. It requires no spraying with poisonous chemicals. The avocado has a perfect balance of life-giving nutrients (potassium, folic acid, fiber, niacin, B6, protein, etc.). It has an unsaturated fat that helps lower LDL "bad" cholesterol. I eat avocados from my Santa Barbara Farm about three times weekly. I mash the avocado, add fresh minced garlic and a dash of Bragg Organic Olive Oil and Bragg Liquid Aminos. I dip slices of tomato, celery, carrot, turnip, cabbage, red onion, cucumber, bell pepper and lettuce leaves into this "guacamole" for a delicious healthy lunch.

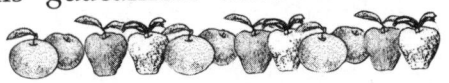

Living under conditions of modern life, it's important to bear in mind that the preparation and refinement of food products either entirely eliminates or in part destroys the vital elements in the original material.
– United States Department of Agriculture - www.usda.gov

Gardenburger Creator Thanks Bragg Books

Paul Wenner, the *Gardenburger* Creator, says his early years as a youth with asthma were so bad he would stand at the window praying to breathe through the night and stay alive. A miracle happened when as a teenager he read the Bragg Books *Miracle of Fasting* and *Bragg Healthy Lifestyle* and his years of asthma were cured in only one month. Paul became so inspired he wanted to be a Health Crusader like Paul Bragg and daughter Patricia – and Paul Wenner has! *Now Gardenburgers are sold worldwide. www.gardenburger.com*

Patricia with Paul Wenner

Foods in a High Health Vibration Contain Life-Giving Substance

When you eat only foods that are in a high health vibration, your body performs and operates by God's Universal Law and becomes a miracle self-starting, self-governing, self-generating instrument! I want you to live by Mother Nature's and God's Laws so your body will be a fine working instrument for a long life. If you have the desire to retain the vitality, energy and enthusiasm of youth and the desire to turn back the clock of Father Time, when your body is bent, your eyes are dimmed and your gait is halting at an age when you should be buoyant with the spirit of youth, then I say:

"There is but one way to live and that is Mother Nature's and God's Healthy Way!"

With Your Hands You Prepare Either Health or Sickness – It's Up to You

They who provide the food for the world, decide the health of the world! A vast multitude of the human race are slaughtered by incompetent cookery. Though you may have taken lessons in music, painting, etc., you are not well-educated unless you have taken lessons in preparing healthy meals. You can either prepare health or sickness with your two hands. Healthy, nutritional planning and preparation produces healthy, delicious meals and healthy bodies.

Juice Fast – Introduction to Water Fast

Fasting has been rediscovered through juice fasting – as a simple, easy means of cleansing and restoring health and vitality. To fast (abstain from food) comes from the Old English word fasten or to hold firm. It's a means to commit oneself to the task of finding inner strength through body, mind and soul cleansing. Throughout history the world's greatest philosophers and sages, including Socrates, Plato, Buddha and Gandhi, have enjoyed fasting and preached its benefits.

Juice bars are springing up everywhere and juice fasting has become "in" with the theatrical crowd in Hollywood, New York and in London. The number of Stars who believe in the power and effectiveness of juice and water fasting is growing. A partial list includes: Steven Spielberg, Barbra Streisand, Kim Basinger, Daryl Hannah, Alec Baldwin, Bette Midler, Christie Brinkley and Cloris Leachman. They say fasting helps balance their lives physically, mentally and emotionally.

Although a pure water fast is best, an introductory liquid juice fast can offer people an ideal opportunity to give their intestinal systems a restful, cleansing relief from the commercial high fat, high sugar, high salt and high protein fast foods too many Americans exist on.

Organic, raw, live fruit and vegetable juices can be purchased fresh from Health Food Stores. You can also prepare these healthy juices yourself using a home juicer. When juice fasting, it's best to dilute juice with $1/3$ distilled water. This list (pg.65) gives you many combination ideas. With vegetable and tomato combinations try adding dash of Bragg Liquid Aminos or Sprinkle or, on non-fast days, even some green powder (alfalfa, barley, chlorella, spirulina, etc.) to create a delicious, nutritious powerful health drink. When using herbs in these drinks, use 1 to 2 fresh leaves or pinch of Bragg Sprinkle (24 herbs & Spices) or pinch of Bragg Kelp (seaweed) rich in protein, iodine and iron – both are delicious with vegetable juices.

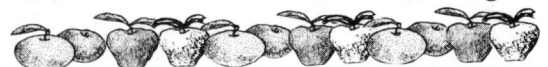

Fasting is the greatest remedy – the physician within!
– Paracelsus, 15th century physician
who established the role of chemistry in medicine

Instead of medicine, fast for a day. – Plutarch, Greek Philosopher

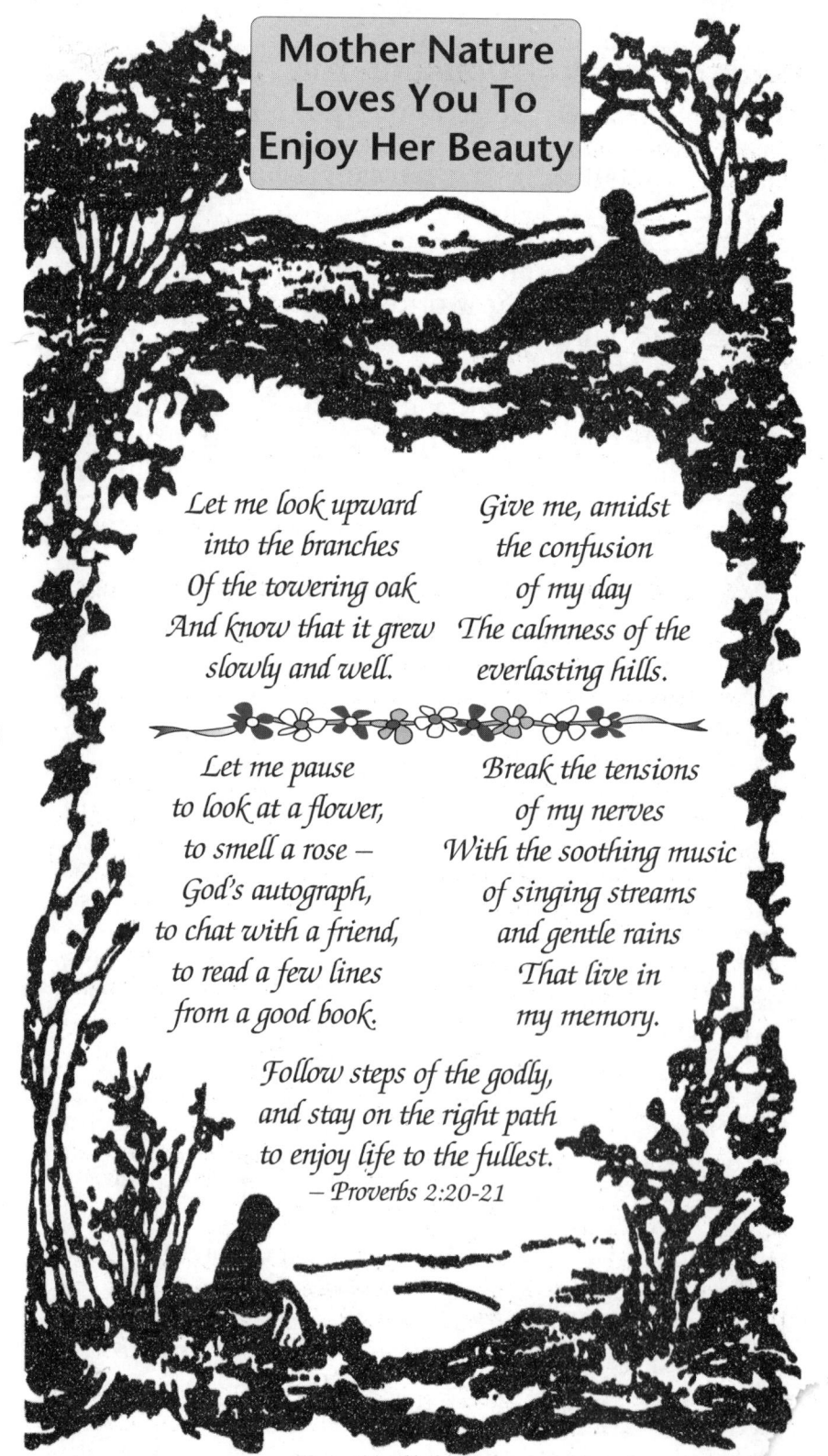

Mother Nature Loves You To Enjoy Her Beauty

Let me look upward
into the branches
Of the towering oak
And know that it grew
slowly and well.

Give me, amidst
the confusion
of my day
The calmness of the
everlasting hills.

Let me pause
to look at a flower,
to smell a rose —
God's autograph,
to chat with a friend,
to read a few lines
from a good book.

Break the tensions
of my nerves
With the soothing music
of singing streams
and gentle rains
That live in
my memory.

Follow steps of the godly,
and stay on the right path
to enjoy life to the fullest.
— Proverbs 2:20-21

64

Open your eyes so you may behold wondrous things out of Thy law. – Psalm 119:18

Powerful Health Combinations to Juice or Blend:

1. Beet, celery, alfalfa sprouts
2. Cabbage, celery and apple
3. Cabbage, cucumber, celery, tomato, spinach and basil
4. Tomato, carrot and celery
5. Carrot, celery, garlic, watercress, goji berries and wheatgrass
6. Grapefruit, orange and lemon
7. Beet, parsley, celery, carrot, mustard greens, cabbage, garlic
8. Beet, celery, kelp and carrot
9. Cucumber, carrot and celery
10. Watercress, apple, cucumber, garlic
11. Asparagus, carrot and apple
12. Carrot, celery, parsley and cabbage, onion, sweet basil
13. Carrot, coconut milk and ginger
14. Carrot, broccoli, lemon, cayenne
15. Carrot, sprouts, kelp, rosemary
16. Apple, carrot, radish, ginger
17. Apple, pineapple and seaweed
18. Apple, papaya and grapes
19. Papaya, cranberries and apple
20. Leafy greens, broccoli, apple
21. Grape, apple and blueberries
22. Watermelon, (seeds optional)

Paul C. Bragg Introduced Juicing to America

Juicing has come a long way since my father imported the first hand operated vegetable-fruit juicer from Germany. Before, this juice was pressed by hand using cheesecloth. He introduced his new juice therapy idea, then pineapple juice, then later tomato juice, to the American public. These two juices were erroneously thought to be too acid. Now, these health beverages have become the favorites of millions. TV's famous *Juicemen* Jack LaLanne and Jay Kordich say Bragg was their early inspiration and mentor! They both are ageless and are still going strong, inspiring millions to health.

65

Fruit bears the closest relation to light. The sun pours a continuous flood of light into fruits. Organic fruits furnish the best food a human being requires for the sustenance of mind and body. – Alcott

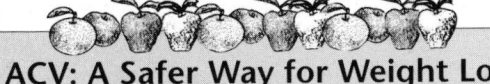

ACV: A Safer Way for Weight Loss

Chemical appetite suppressants and diet aids are flooding the market! Many have caused serious health problems, even death! Millions are searching for more natural ways to lose unwanted pounds and many are looking at Apple Cider Vinegar. The pectin found in apples is one of the benefits attributed to the correlation between ACV and weight loss. Pectin, a natural fiber, helps clean out the digestive tract, plus, the acidic nature of ACV helps stimulate a bodily response that burns stored fat that accelerates weight loss!

Deeds of kindness, smiles and little words of love and thanks help to make people and earth happy, like Heaven above. – Julia Carney

Caution: The Army Diet – what you overeat goes to the front.

Liquefied and Fresh Juiced Foods

The juicer, food processor and blender are great for preparing foods for gentle or bland diets and baby foods. Fibers of fresh fruits and vegetables juiced can be tolerated on most gentle diets. Any raw or cooked fruit or vegetable can be liquefied and added to non-dairy milks - soy, rice, nut, almond, etc., or broth or soups. Live, fresh juices super charge your body's health power! You may fortify your liquid meal with barley green, alfalfa, chlorella, soy, spirulina, and vitamin C powder for extra super nutrition.

The Bragg Healthy Lifestyle Promotes Super Health and Longevity

The Bragg Healthy Lifestyle consists of eating a diet of 60% to 70% fresh, live, organically grown foods; raw vegetables, salads, fresh fruits and juices; sprouts, raw seeds and nuts; all-natural 100% whole-grain breads, pastas, cereals and nutritious beans and legumes. These are the no cholesterol, no fat, no salt, "live foods" which combine to make up the body fuel that creates healthy, lively people that want to exercise and be fit. This healthy diet also creates energy. This is the reason people become revitalized and reborn into a fresh new life filled with joy, health, vitality, youthfulness and longevity! There are millions of healthy Bragg followers around the world proving that this Bragg Healthy Lifestyle works!

Pure Water is Important for Health

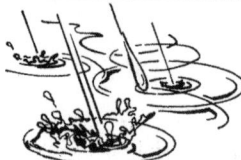

To the days of the aged, it addeth length;
To the might of the strong, it addeth strength;
It freshens the heart, it brightens the sight;
It's like drinking a goblet of morning light.

The body is 70% water and purified, steam-distilled (chemical-free) water is important for total health. You should drink 8-10 glasses of water a day. Read our revealing book, *Water – The Shocking Truth That Can Save Your Life,* for info on importance of purified water (pages 120, 127).

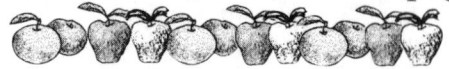

Drinking 8-10 glasses daily of pure distilled water cleanses and recharges the human batteries! – Paul C. Bragg, N.D., Ph.D.

Be Safe – Drink Purified, Distilled Water!

Pure distilled water is vitally important in following The Bragg Healthy Heart Lifestyle. Water is the key to all body functions including: digestion, assimilation, elimination and circulation, and to bones and joints, muscles, nerves, glands and senses. The right kind of water is one of your best natural protections against all kinds of diseases and infections. It's a vital factor in all the body fluids, tissues, cells, lymph, blood and all glandular secretions. Water holds all nutritive factors in solution, as well as toxins and body wastes, and acts as the main transportation medium throughout the body, for both nutrition and cleansing purposes (pg. 33).

Since your body is about 70% water, the blood and lymphatic system is over 90% water, it's essential for your health that you drink only pure water that's not saturated with contaminants, inorganic minerals and toxins. This pure water will transport vital nutrients to cells and waste from cells more efficiently. This allows the body to function correctly and stay healthier!

ORGANIC MINERALS Your minerals must come from an organic source, from something living or that has lived. Humans do not have the same chemistry as plants. Only the living plant has the ability to extract inorganic minerals from the earth and convert them to organic minerals for your body to absorb and utilize.

INORGANIC MINERALS Inorganic minerals and toxic chemicals in water can create these problems:

- *Causes arthritis, bone spurs and painful calcified formations in the joints.*
- *Hardens the liver.*
- *Causes kidney and gallstones.*
- *Clogs and hardens the veins, capillaries and arteries.*
- *Inorganic minerals and the toxic chemicals in water, clog the arteries and small capillaries that are needed to feed and nourish your brain with oxygenated blood; the result is gradual loss of memory and senility and strokes.*

Cocktail of Toxic Chemicals

Chlorine, fluoride, calcium carbonate cadmium, aluminum, trihalomethanes, chloroform, arsenic copper, lead and unpleasant taste

Tap-Water Average Contents

Water is the key to all body functions including: digestion, circulation, bones and joints, assimilation, elimination, muscles, nerves, glands and the senses.

Skin Absorbs Water, Toxins and All

From the American Journal of Public Health - www.ajph.org

Compared with its vast absorption through the respiratory system, skin absorption could be the major route of penetration into the body. Skin penetration rates have been found to be remarkably high, and the outer layer of skin is a less effective barrier to penetration than traditionally assumed. Factors affecting absorption are:

Hydration: The more hydrated the skin, the greater the absorption. If the skin is hydrated by perspiration or immersion in water or if the contaminant compounds are in solution, penetration is enhanced.

Temperature: Increased skin or water temperature will enhance skin absorption capacity proportionately. During swimming and bathing, it may be expected that greater hydration of skin surfaces will take place.

Skin Condition: Any insult (i.e. sunburn) or injury (i.e. cuts, wounds, abrasions) to the skin will lower its ability to act as a barrier against foreign substances. A history of skin disease such as psoriasis or eczema acts to lower the natural barrier of the outer skin layer, as do rashes, dermatitis, or any chronic skin condition.

Regional Variability: Skin absorption rates vary with the different regions of the body. Underestimated is the case of whole body immersion during swimming or bathing. The epidermis of the hand represents a relatively greater barrier to penetration than many other parts of the body, including the scalp, forehead, abdomen, area in and around the ears, underarms and genital area. Penetration through the genital area is estimated to be 100%, but only 8.6% for the forearm.

Other Routes of Entry: Other routes of absorption include oral, nasal, cheeks and mouth cavity, and eye and ear areas. These routes have been underestimated in their ability to absorb contaminants during immersion in water. Inhalation serves as yet another route. In the case of swimming or bathing, the volatilized chemicals are likely to gather near the surface of the water and are readily inhalable. In addition, some may be swallowed.

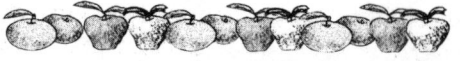

You Get More Toxic Exposure from Taking a Chlorinated Water Shower Than From Drinking the Same Water!

Two of the very highly toxic and volatile chemicals, trichloroethylene and chloroform, have been proven as toxic contaminants found in most all municipal drinking water supplies. The National Academy of Sciences recently has estimated that hundreds of people die in the United States each year from the cancers caused largely by ingesting water pollutants from inhalation as air pollutants in the home. Inhalation exposure to water pollutants is largely ignored. Recent shocking data indicates that hot showers can liberate about 50% of the chloroform and 80% of the trichloroethylene into the air.

Tests show your body can absorb more toxic chlorine from a 10-minute shower than drinking 8 glasses of the same water. How can that be? A warm shower opens up your pores, causing your skin to act like a sponge. As a result, you not only inhale the chlorine vapors, you also absorb them through your skin, directly into your bloodstream – at a rate that's up to 6 times higher than drinking it.

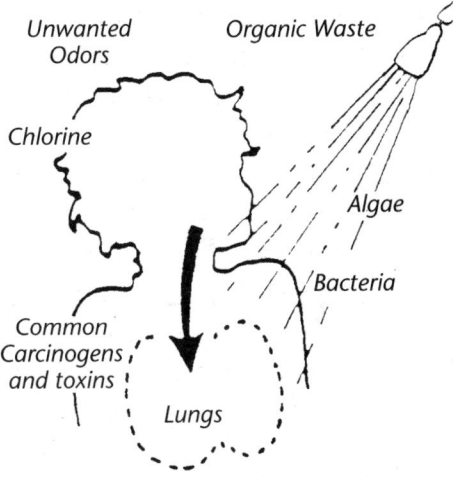

" In terms of cumulative damage to your health, showering in chlorinated water is one of the most dangerous risks you take daily. Short-term risks include: eyes, sinus, throat, skin and lung irritation. Long-term risks include: excessive free radical formation (that ages you!) higher vulnerability to genetic mutation and cancer development; and difficulty metabolizing cholesterol, causing hardened arteries".
– Science News - www.sciencenews.org

The treatment of diseases should go to the root cause, and most often it is found in severe dehydration from lack of sufficient pure, distilled water, plus an unhealthy lifestyle! See web for important info: www.watercure.com.

69

Five Hidden Toxic Dangers in Your Shower:

● **Chlorine:** Added to all municipal water supplies, this disinfectant hardens arteries, destroys cells and tissues, irritates skin, sinus conditions and aggravates asthma, allergies and respiratory problems. *www.bidness.com/esd/showering.htm*

● **Chloroform:** This powerful by-product of chlorination causes excessive free radical formation (a cause of accelerated ageing!), normal cells to mutate and cholesterol to form. It's a known carcinogen!

● **DCA (Dichloroacedic acid):** This chlorine by-product alters cholesterol metabolism and has been shown to cause liver cancer in lab animals.

● **MX (toxic chlorinated acid):** Another by-product of chlorination, MX is known to cause genetic mutations that can lead to cancer growth and has been found in all chlorinated water for which it was tested.

● **Cause of bladder and rectal cancer:** Research proved chlorinated water is direct cause of over 9% of U.S. bladder cancers, 15% of rectal cancers and rise in heart disease.

70

Showers, Toxic Chemicals & Chlorine

Skin absorption of toxic contaminants has been underestimated and ingestion may not constitute sole or even primary route of exposure. – Dr. Halina Brown *– American Journal of Public Health, – www.ajph.org*

Taking long hot showers is a health risk, according to latest research. Showers can lead to greater exposure to toxic chemicals contained in the water supplies than does drinking the water. These toxic chemicals evaporate out of the water and are inhaled. They can also spread through the house and be inhaled by others. People receive 6 to 100 times more chemicals by breathing the air around showers and baths than they would by drinking the water. *– www. newscientist.com*

A University of Pittsburgh Professor of Water Chemistry claims that exposure to vaporized chemicals in the water supplies through showering, bathing and inhalation is 100 times greater than through drinking the water. *– The Nader Report – Troubled Waters on Tap, – nader.org*

The power of pure water is the vital chemistry of life.

Chlorine in the water is the greatest crippler and killer of modern times. While it prevented epidemics of one disease, it was creating another. 20 years after the start of chlorinating drinking water in 1904, the present epidemic of heart trouble, cancer and senility began. – Dr. Joseph Price, author, *Coronaries/Cholesterol/Chlorine*

Don't Gamble – Use a Shower Filter

The most effective method of removing hazards from your shower is the quick and easy installation of a filter on your shower arm. We use a good filter that removes chlorine, lead, mercury, iron, arsenic, hydrogen sulfide, and many other unseen contaminants, such as bacteria, fungi, dirt and sediments. With a 12-18 month life-span, this filter is easily cleaned by backwashing every 2-3 months and is replaceable. So start enjoying safe, chlorine-free showers. It reduces risk of heart disease and cancer and the strain on your immune system. You may even get rid of long-standing conditions, from sinus, respiratory problems to dry, itchy skin. To order this shower filter – weekdays call 800-446-1990. We use this filter and am thankful for chlorine-free showers!

Bragg's Vinegar Eye Wash for Cataracts

My 70 year-young gardener in California went to his eye doctor because his eyes were getting cloudy. He was told he needed cataract surgery! Then he began drinking our vinegar drink and using Bragg's Vinegar Eye Wash. Now his eyes are perfectly clear and he's seeing better than ever!

Police Captain Diane's best friend Spike is $14^1/2$. His eyes were becoming increasingly more clouded by cataracts. Diane began using Bragg's Vinegar Eye Wash in his eyes and now they are crystal clear and Spike is a happy doggie!

Bragg's Vinegar Eye Wash:

$1/3$ tsp Bragg Apple Cider Vinegar in 4 oz. distilled water. You can use as an eyewash or as drops. Repeat 2 to 3 times daily. Keep eye lids closed for 2 minutes after applying liquid. Sometimes slight smarting occurs.

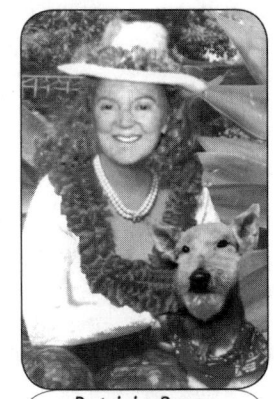

Patricia Bragg with clear-eyed Spike

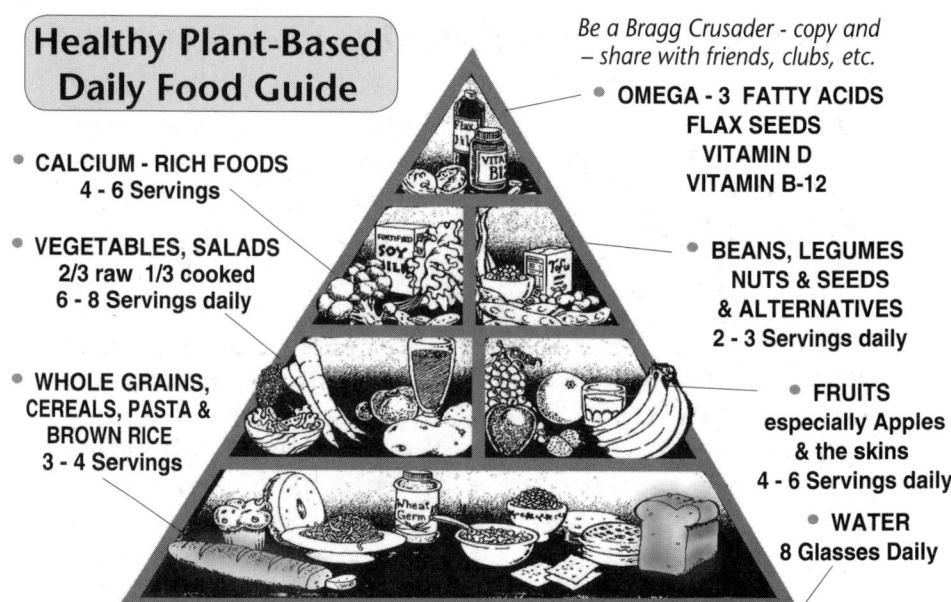

Healthy Plant-Based Daily Food Guide

Be a Bragg Crusader - copy and – share with friends, clubs, etc.

- OMEGA - 3 FATTY ACIDS
  FLAX SEEDS
  VITAMIN D
  VITAMIN B-12

- CALCIUM - RICH FOODS
  4 - 6 Servings

- VEGETABLES, SALADS
  2/3 raw 1/3 cooked
  6 - 8 Servings daily

- BEANS, LEGUMES
  NUTS & SEEDS
  & ALTERNATIVES
  2 - 3 Servings daily

- WHOLE GRAINS,
  CEREALS, PASTA &
  BROWN RICE
  3 - 4 Servings

- FRUITS
  especially Apples
  & the skins
  4 - 6 Servings daily

- WATER
  8 Glasses Daily

8 Glasses Daily Purified/Distilled Water

Warning! – Avoid All Unhealthy Microwaved Foods!

In the past 25 years (health destroying) microwaves have practically replaced traditional methods of cooking, especially with on-the-go people of today's world. But how much do you really know about them? Are they no more than timesaving machines for cooking? A Swiss Study found that food which is microwaved is not the food it was before! The microwave radiation deforms and destroys the molecular structure of the food – creating radiolytic compounds! When microwaved food is eaten, abnormal changes occur in the blood and immune systems. These include a decrease in hemoglobin and white blood cell counts and an increase in cholesterol levels. An article in Pediatrics Journal warns microwaving human milk damages the anti-infective properties it usually gives to a mother's baby. Recent work being done University of Warwick in Great Britain warns that microwave radiation is damaging to the vital electromagnetic activity of human life vibrations. Over 20 years ago Russia established wise microwave radiation limits more stringent than United States and Great Britain. Beware don't use microwaves!! See web: relfe.com/microwave.html

Aspartame – Artificial Diet Sweetener Unhealthy & Makes You Fat!

Because Monsanto's artificial sweetener Aspartame (sold as "Nutrasweet," "Equal," & "Spoonful") is over 200 times sweeter than sugar, it's a common ingredient found in "diet" foods and has become a sweetening staple for dieters. Besides being a deadly poison, aspartame actually contributes to weight gain by causing a craving for carbohydrates. A study of 80,000 women by American Cancer Society found those who used this neurotoxic "diet" sweetener actually gained more weight than those who didn't use aspartame products. Find out more about the deadly health risks posed by Monsanto's toxic sweetener on this web: aspartamekills.com/lydon.htm. Stevia, an herbal sweetener is a healthy alternative for diabetics.

Exercise is Vital for Health & Longevity

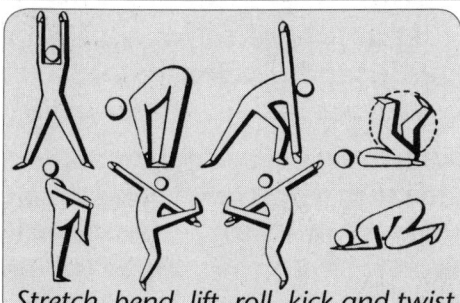

Stretch, bend, lift, roll, kick and twist

To ensure youthful arteries, exercise is very essential! If you wish to live and enjoy a long, fit and healthy life it's necessary to build up your cardiovascular endurance and start to follow an exercise program designed to keep your arteries unclogged, soft, agile and healthy. The first step is to get more oxygen into the body which will help dissolve the encrustations that have formed in the arteries. Any physical activity that injects more oxygen is going to help extend your life!

Enjoy a Tireless – Ageless – Pain-free Body as Conrad Hilton, J.C. Penney & Dr. Scholl did With The Bragg Healthy Lifestyle

Don't despair in your golden years – enjoy them! My dad Paul C. Bragg, said *life's second half is the best* and can be the most healthy fruitful years. Linus Pauling, painter Grandma Moses and amazing Mother Teresa, have all proven that! These three famous Bragg health followers – Conrad Hilton, J.C. Penney and foot Dr. Scholl – all lived strong, productive, active lives to almost 100 years. Countless others have lived long, healthy fulfilled lives following The Bragg Healthy Lifestyle, you can too!

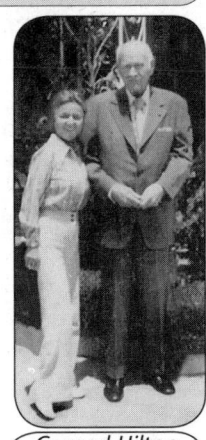

Conrad Hilton with Patricia

73

We teach you how to forget calendar years and to regain not only a youthful spirit, but much of the vigor of your youth. It's your duty to yourself to start to live The Bragg Healthy Lifestyle today – don't procrastinate! Keep premature ageing out of your body by faithfully living this healthy lifestyle blueprint. You must eat foods that have a high health vibration rate (abundance of raw, organic fruits and vegetables) and do a water fast weekly.

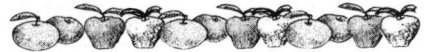

It's never too late to get into shape, but it does take daily perseverance.
– Dr. Thomas K. Cureton – Physical Fitness Pioneer, University of Illinois

Also, do some Bragg Super Power Deep Breathing exercises, get 8 hours of restful sleep at night and keep your body relaxed. Don't let anything rob you of your emotional and nervous energy and precious vital force! Do read *Bragg Powerful Nerve Force and Breathing Books*.

Your body is being made anew every day! Premature ageing and senility result from the toxic debris that accumulates when you live an unhealthy lifestyle. Eat right, exercise for good body circulation, and there will be little or no buildup of toxins to clog and prematurely age your body. Cultivate and hold onto the spirit of youth *and it will be yours!* You can feel and look younger! Keep your spine straight to maintain high energy level. Daily do The Bragg Posture Exercise on page 80. Follow The Bragg Healthy Lifestyle and you will be blessed with many miracles!

If you are already in the clutches of premature ageing, begin now to fight for the return of youth. Work to restore this priceless possession! You can do it! Train your body as you would that of a race horse. Follow these clear, definite instructions and you will gain strength, virility, energy, vivacity and enthusiasm! Make your life a daily enjoyment of the most precious of all earthly gifts – the power and joys of youthful, healthful living. Men and women can be young at 60, 70, 80 and even 90 (pages 9, 88-90). Some have retained the spirit of youth beyond the century mark, like the Hunzas of Kashmir and Georgians of Russia are still doing!

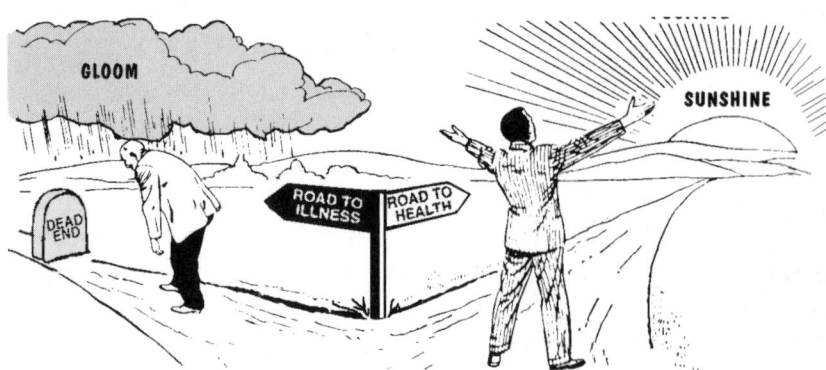

NEGATIVE ← OR → POSITIVE
The choice of which road to take is up to you.

You alone decide whether to reach a dead end or live a healthy lifestyle for a long, healthy, happy, active life. – Paul C. Bragg

The three greatest letters in the English alphabet are N-O-W. There is no time like the present. Begin Now! – Sir Walter Scott, Scottish Poet, 18th C.

Health Suggestions for Your Daily Program

Those of you who live the incomplete life, and give up the precious qualities of human existence for dietary excesses or for the pleasures of luxury and idleness, are selling your birthright for a mess of pottage! Wake up to the possibilities within your reach! Rejuvenate your body. Make your mind keen and capable. Obey the Laws of Mother Nature and God and you will see results that you now scarcely dare to dream! Miracles will happen!

Be sure that you sleep in a well ventilated, uncluttered, dust-free room, so you get a large amount of clean oxygen while sleeping. I know it's often difficult to keep dust collectors (knick-knacks, etc.) out of your home. We recently had to unclutter some areas due to dust mites. It's best to vacuum carpets often, using a hepa filter or a micro-liner bag. Put pillows and mattresses (dust mites' haven) in protective zip-closed covers. Make sure your mattress is firm, flat (have head elevated on pillow), also try 2" memory foam topper. Sleep spread-out to allow for good circulation. It's best not to sleep in cramped position or sleep on your arms.

Oxygen is The Invisible Staff of Life

Oxygen is the life of the blood, and blood is the life of the body! A person weighing about 150 pounds contains about 88 pounds of oxygen. Oxygen is the most important element in the body. It is colorless, odorless and tasteless. Its main function is purification. Lack of oxygen in the body can lead to serious consequences. The majority of people are oxygen starved because they are shallow breathers. Do read *our Bragg Super Power Breathing* book.

To have a healthy, youthful, vital life, we need fresh, unpolluted air in abundance, pure distilled water and plenty of fresh organic vegetables and fruits. Remember, oxygen is an unquestionable source of indispensable energy necessary for higher vital activity in the human organism! It helps ensure healthier elimination, reconstruction and regeneration within the vital factors and metabolic activities of the entire physical body.

The body is self-cleansing and self-healing! It is our duty if we want vibrant, glorious health, to do all we can to make the body work efficiently to maintain vital, super health. Not only is a healthy diet necessary, but so are good sleeping habits, outdoor physical activity, full, deep breathing and a serene, peaceful mind. We cannot live by bread alone. We must have spiritual food. And also strive for a perfect healthy balance: physical, mental, emotional and spiritual!

Through the lung functioning, oxygen is absorbed and assimilated into the bloodstream, bringing with it other unknown factors from the atmosphere. Plants, through their roots, absorb the vital elements in the soil necessary for their life. If we cut or damage their roots, they die! Man's roots are his lungs. Smokers are killing their lungs and the lungs of all those around them! Don't be around secondhand smoke – it's even more deadly! Allow no smoking in your home! See web *bragg.com* for the dangers of smoking from the *Bragg Breathing Book*.

We can only breathe adequately with sufficient physical movement. With the proper movements we are motivated to obtain the full elixir of life which is the breath of air. The stronger and more vigorous our movements, the more air we need and the deeper we breathe.

The oxygen in the air that we breathe helps dissolve and eliminate waste and builds the continuum of our cellular structure, thus maintaining our body to the highest degree possible! Each breath should detoxify and regenerate our vital forces. But this rejuvenation process must be supplemented by faithfully following The Bragg Healthy Lifestyle. Please understand that both exercise and deep breathing must be fortified with proper healthy nutrition to prevent the degenerative and destructive premature breakdown of the cells.

This explains why there is a physical decline in top athletes in their late 20s who haven't consumed a correct nutritionally, balanced diet. The average athlete reaches a peak at about 27 and then, sadly, begins to decline! I know this to be true, as my father was an active athlete his whole life and we saw the finest athletes reach their peak and then slowly decline, and sad to say many of them dying way too young.

Other factors affecting breathing: Our thoughts and emotions interfere with our breathing. That's why, if we have a headache or some other sudden symptom, a few minutes of deep breathing exercises in the open air will help us detoxify and reestablish our internal balance.

Actress Cloris Leachman is an ardent health follower who sparkles with health. She hates smoking, coffee, alcohol, sugar and meat. One of her solutions to health problems is to fast. "Fasting is a miracle cure. It cured my asthma."

To Rest is to Rust and Rust is Destruction!

Upon waking in the morning, stretch your legs, arms and body as you do when yawning. Continue this stretching process until you feel that every muscle has been properly and fully awakened. Good circulation and elimination are the master keys to good health! That is the reason it is important to stretch and exercise your body. Don't restrict your exercises to the morning. Make some time for them during the day to keep your circulation strong throughout your cardiovascular system during all your waking hours. Don't sit longer than one hour at a time. Do some stretching and deep breathing exercises. Get up and move around. Don't sit in a car for more than two hours. Stop the car, get out and stretch and exercise your legs and body (see exercises page 73 & 80).

Exercises Will Help Keep You More Healthy, Youthful, Flexible and Fit

You must fight off stiffness if you want the body to feel youthful. Most prematurely old people find it impossible to straighten their spines or continually maintain good posture. Why? Because their bodies have become stiff and rigid through lack of exercise and use. It is no wonder that men and women become prematurely old, settle down and get crusty and stiff-necked. They don't do exercises that move their spinal joints! If you have already begun to acquire this stiffness, take warning now and reverse old age habits! It's never too late!

An Old English Prayer

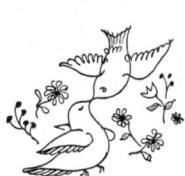

Give us Lord, a bit of sun,
A bit of work and a bit of fun.
Give us, in all struggle and sputter,
Our daily whole grain bread and food.
Give us health, our keep to make
And a bit to spare for others' sake.
Give us too, a bit of song
And a tale and a book, to help us along.
Give us Lord, a chance to be
Our goodly best for ourselves and others
Until men learn to live as brothers.

Through our actions and deeds, rather than promises,
let us display the essence of love – perfect harmony in motion!
– Philip Glyn, Welsh Poet

Keep Your Spine Flexible and Youthful

Go to work on yourself! One of the main keys to looking 10 years younger is to keep your spine active, so strive for flexibility and elasticity in every part of your body, especially your spine! Also, remember to stand, walk and sit tall because all youthful-looking people have good posture.

The spine is a marvelous instrument as well as the central support of the whole body. It is made up of a flexible column of squarish bones that are joined together with rubbery puffs called discs. This wonderful piece of equipment stores its own lubrication in little sacs at the joints. The spine was designed for action! Keep it loose and supple, and your whole body will move with grace, ease and youthfulness. Read the *Bragg Back Fitness Program* Book for the Bragg Simple Spine Exercises to help keep your spine and you flexible and youthful.

Your Waist-Line is Your Life-Line, Date-Line and Health-Line!

Get a tape measure and measure your waist. Write down the measurement. If you consciously pursue vigorous abdominal and postural exercises combined with correct eating and a weekly 24 hour fast (and later on, 3 to 7 day fasts), in a short time you'll see a more trim and youthful waist-line! Trim waist-lines can make people appear years younger. Now, let's get yours down to where it should be, if it has grown too big and fat. It's a trim, lean horse for the long race of life! I'm sure we all want longevity! Studies show *the bigger the waist-line – the shorter the life-span*. Living The Bragg Healthy Lifestyle is so wonderful. Your life and each day is a precious gift to enjoy, treasure and guard.

People abuse their abdomens abominably! You cannot eat dead, empty-calorie foods and tell yourself that a tiny snack here and there won't show! You are completely wrong! Dead, devitalized foods create toxic poisons inside your body and this all helps to add flabby unhealthy fat and inches to your abdomen and body.

Nothing transforms a person faster than changing from a negative to a positive attitude.
– Paul C. Bragg N.D., Ph.D., Originator of Health Food Stores

Large Waist-Lines Lead to Shorter Life-Spans

Do not overeat even healthy foods, for your body only needs enough food (fuel) to maintain health and energy. People become overweight because they have over-fueled their bodies. Studies show large waist-lines produce shorter lifespans. Visit web: *www.obesity.org*

You are not getting away with this kind of cheating, you are just cheating (hurting) yourself! Bear in mind that as we live longer, the internal abdominal structure and stomach muscles relax more. This is called droopy tummy or visceroptosis. It's a common condition among older people who don't exercise their waist muscles. It can be a contributing cause of constipation, sluggish liver and even hernias. (Start Bragg Posture Exercise, page 80.)

When the abdominal wall becomes lazy and the consequent droop is compounded by fatty layers of flab, then trouble starts inside the abdomen. By the time most people reach 40, they have a prolapsed abdomen. Become a people watcher and you will notice that what I'm saying is true! Some need a surgical tummy-tuck (which removes excess flab) to give them a flat stomach. So, don't let your abdominal muscles droop! Make every effort to recapture firmness. It's amazing how quickly muscles respond to exercises, sit-ups and good posture.

Maintain Youthful Posture for Super-Health

There is a fundamental relationship between good posture and youth on the one hand and between bent posture and age on the other! To maintain the posture of youth actually means to maintain youth itself, because of the basic relationship between the healthy, normal spine and bodily vigor: the condition that signifies youth, irrespective of how many years one has lived.

The most easily recognized sign of premature ageing is the forward bending of the spine, combined with the "rounded shoulders" that accompany it. Prematurely old people often exhibit this condition to an extreme degree, almost bending over double. Even some school children sometimes display early signs of premature ageing . . .

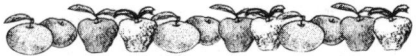

We can change and improve if we set our will to improve. – Robert Benson

poor posture, stooped, rounded shoulders, and sunken-in chests! On the other hand, people of advanced years, by simply straightening their spines and walking more erect, appear 10 to 30 years younger than they really are. Look around you – start noticing postures of all ages and you will see what I mean! Dad and I enjoy posture watching.

One's entire life must be a constant fight to maintain the correct, erect posture, for this then gives your heart and internal organs room to operate more efficiently. Remember, the spine is the fundamental structure of the body. Along with the brain, the spine constitutes the center of the nervous system. All other parts of the body are, so to speak, appendages of the spine. Keep that spinal column straight, keep it flexible and youthful! Good health and longevity depend on a healthy, erect body. Never cross your legs – sit tall with both feet on floor. Stretch up your spine to sit, stand and walk tall. Check your body and posture (best in bathing suit or nude) in the mirror. See where you are on the posture chart – perfect, fair or poor? Start improving from today on!

Bragg Posture Exercise Gives Youthfulness

Before a mirror, stand up, feet 8" apart, stretch up spine. Tighten buttocks and suck in stomach muscles, lift up rib cage, put chest out, shoulders back, and chin up slightly. Line body up straight (nose plumbline straight to belly button), drop hands to sides and swing arms to normalize your posture. Do this posture exercise faithfully daily and miraculous changes will happen! You are retraining and strengthening your muscles to stand straight for health and youthfulness. Remember when you slump, you also cramp your precious machinery. This posture exercise will retrain your frame to sit, stand and walk tall for supreme health and longevity!

Posture improves with massages – soothing, relaxing and brings beneficial healthy changes, improves circulation help unclog the body forces which then promotes more healing and smoother, more fit muscles. See pgs. 91 to 94.

A strong body makes the mind strong. – Thomas Jefferson, 3rd U.S. President

I like the laughter that opens the lips and the heart, that shows at the same time the pearls and the soul. – Victor Hugo

WHERE DO YOU STAND?

POSTURE CHART

	PERFECT	FAIR	POOR
HEAD			
SHOULDERS			
SPINE			
HIPS			
ANKLES			
NECK			
UPPER BACK			
TRUNK			
ABDOMEN			
LOWER BACK			

81

Your posture carries you through life from your head to your feet. This is your human vehicle and you are truly a miracle! Cherish, respect and always protect it by living The Bragg Healthy Lifestyle. – Patricia Bragg

The strongest principles of growth lies in human choice. – George Eliot

Remember – Your posture can make or break your health!

Stop Dying – Start Healthy Living Now!
The Bible tells us that . . .
The kingdom of Heaven is within us.

I thoroughly believe this statement! We can make this body we live in either a kingdom of heaven on earth or we can make it a torture chamber. It's all up to you! After childhood, the kind of body you live in is strictly up to you! I cannot live your life for you! Nor can anyone else! You are a mature adult, and you must face the realities of life. I am sure you have the willpower and desire to follow The Bragg Healthy Lifestyle, so start now on the road to Higher Health – start today!

This is the Bragg Master Blueprint to greater physical perfection because it works with the Laws of God and Mother Nature, and they make no compromises! You either follow them or they break you! You can't break a Natural Law or God Law, for it will break you in time!

Natural Health Laws for Physical Perfection
These Natural Laws God and Mother Nature put in motion are wise, perfect laws created for your own good:

- *You must eat natural foods and never overeat.*
- *You must breathe deeply of God's pure air.*
- *You must exercise the 640 muscles of your body.*
- *You must give your body pure, safe, clean water.*
- *You must give your body gentle sunshine.*
- *You must not overwork or burden your body; this leads to stress, tensions and nerve depletion.*
- *You must keep the body clean inside and outside.*
- *You must live by divine intelligence and wisdom.*

The human body is a miracle, give it the best. Within us is the inherent potential to become perfect! It is the intent of our Creator for us to have a physically perfect, healthy, happy and peaceful long life! – *Genesis 6:3*

Making positive lifestyle changes – daily exercise, healthy eating, eliminating stress and educating yourself about heart disease – lowers heart disease risk.
– Johns Hopkins Medical News • www.hopkinsmedicine.org

With every new day comes new strength and new thoughts. – Eleanor Roosevelt

Enjoy Mother Nature's and God's Foods

When we are not physically perfect, we are out of harmony with the Creator's design, and therefore out of harmony with God's intent, will and law (3 John 2). In simpler words, we are, in our unhealthy living habits, opposing the will of God and Mother Earth. So, you see that to reach physical perfection, we must live correctly on all four important planes: the physical, the mental, the emotional and the spiritual. By living on the physical plane correctly, we can then reach a higher mental, emotional and spiritual state for perfection.

If you eat God's and Mother Nature's Foods and build a healthy, clean bloodstream, you are going to be keener mentally. The wonderful part of living by this blueprint is that we find a new calmness coming over us. You'll experience a new feeling of confidence, peace, joy and serenity! When every cell, organ and body part is functioning perfectly, the body becomes more perfect physically, mentally, emotionally and spiritually. What complete satisfaction you will feel when you are living The Bragg Healthy Lifestyle and reaping the great rewards of a healthier, happier, stronger and more fulfilled life!

Your degree of physical perfection is the measure of your efforts in cooperating by daily partaking of proper foods, exercise, deep breathing and youthful thinking. This is your Creator's health design and intent so that you can become strong and remain physically healthy, youthful, active and of service, regardless of your age! Four exemplary long lives of devoted service we admire: Albert Einstein, Gandhi, Albert Schweitzer, Mother Teresa.

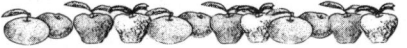

Thousands of people every year pay thousands of dollars for state-of-the-art testing to learn their risk for heart disease. However, experts say that fresh vegetables and a health club membership may be better buys than any lab test. People who eat a diet low in fat and cholesterol and rich in plant foods, who don't smoke, who exercise regularly, and keep their weight and blood pressure in the normal range are less likely to have a heart attack than those who don't despite any predisposition or genetic tendency toward heart disease.
– Harvard Health Letter • www.health.harvard.edu

Spread love everywhere you go: first of all in your own house. Give love to your children, to your wife or husband, to a next door neighbor . . . Let no one ever come to you without leaving better and happier. Be the living expression of God's kindness; kindness in your face, kindness in your eyes, kindness in your smile and kindness in your warm greeting. – Mother Teresa

Food and Product Summary

Today, many of our foods are highly processed or refined, robbing them of essential nutrients, vitamins, minerals and enzymes. Many also contain harmful, toxic and dangerous chemicals. The research findings and experience of top nutritionists, physicians and dentists have led to the discovery that devitalized foods are a major cause of poor health, illness, cancer and premature death. The enormous increase in the last 70 years of degenerative diseases such as heart disease, arthritis and dental decay substantiate this belief. Scientific research has shown that most of these afflictions can be prevented and others, once established, can be arrested or even reversed through nutritional methods (pages 7, 19, 79).

Enjoy Super Health with Natural Foods

1. **RAW FOODS:** Fresh fruits and raw vegetables organically grown are always best! Enjoy nutritious variety garden salads with raw vegetables, greens, sprouts, raw nuts and seeds.

2. **VEGETABLES and PROTEINS:**
   a. Legumes, lentils, brown rice, soy beans, and all beans.
   b. Nuts and seeds, raw and unsalted.
   c. We prefer healthier vegetarian proteins. If you must have animal protein, then be sure it's hormone-free, and organically fed and no more than 1 or 2 times a week.
   d. Dairy products – fertile range-free eggs (*not over 4 weekly*), unprocessed hard cheese and feta goat's cheese. We choose not to use dairy products! Try healthier non-dairy soy, rice, nut, and almond milks and soy cheeses, delicious soy yogurt and the soy and rice ice creams.

3. **FRUITS and VEGETABLES:** Organically grown is always best – grown without the use of poisonous sprays and toxic chemical fertilizers whenever possible; urge your market to stock organic produce! Steam, bake, sauté and wok vegetables as short a time as possible to retain the best nutritional content and flavor. Also enjoy fresh juices.

4. **100% WHOLE GRAIN CEREALS, BREADS and FLOURS:** They contain important B-complex vitamins, vitamin E, minerals, fiber and the important unsaturated fatty acids.

5. **COLD or EXPELLER-PRESSED VEGETABLE OILS:** Bragg Organic extra virgin Olive Oil (is best), soy, sunflower, flax and sesame oils are excellent sources of healthy, essential, unsaturated fatty acids. We still use oils sparingly.

84

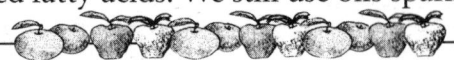

USA leads world in obesity, heart disease, strokes, cancer and diabetes! Why? It's our fast junk foods, high sugars, meats, fats, dairy and processed foods diet.

The Body Must Obey Your Strong, Wise Mind

Flesh is dumb! You can put anything in your stomach from coffee to hot dogs. It is not the stomach that rules the body, but your intelligent and reasoning mind! Let me close The Bragg Healthy Lifestyle Blueprint with the unequivocal statement that the properly-directed mind can inspire the body to follow this Blueprint, thereby helping the body to become closer to physical perfection.

Morning Resolve To Start Your Day

I will this day live a simple, sincere and serene life; repelling promptly every thought of impurity, discontent, anxiety, fear, and discouragement. I will cultivate health, cheerfulness, happiness, charity and the love of brotherhood; exercising economy in expenditure, generosity in giving, carefulness in conversation and diligence in appointed service. I pledge fidelity to every trust and a childlike faith in God. I will be faithful in those habits of prayer, study, work, nutrition, physical exercise, deep breathing and good posture. I shall fast for a 24 hour period each week, eat only healthy foods and get sufficient sleep each night. I will make every effort to improve myself physically, mentally, emotionally and spiritually every day.

Morning Prayer used by Patricia Bragg and her father, Paul C. Bragg

Dear Friend, I wish above all things that thou may prosper and be in health even as the soul prospers. – 3 John 2

This is God's and Our Goal for You – Radiant, Super Health! – 3 John 2

Hippocrates, Aristotle, Galen, Paracelsus, Plato, Socrates and other great philosophers, scientists and physicians for centuries have used fasting as a method of cleansing, healing and renewing the body, physically & spiritually.

Avoid all self-drugging, such as aspirin and similar drugs, pain-killers, sleeping pills, tranquilizers, antihistamines, laxatives, strong cathartics and fizzing bromides, etc. You are not qualified to prescribe drugs for yourself, and the side-effects and results can be serious. – Patricia Bragg, N.D.,Ph.D. Health Crusader

Anyone who stops learning is old, whether 20 or 80. Anyone who keeps learning stays youthful. The greatest thing in life is to keep your mind young. – Henry Ford

The doctor of the future will give no medicine, but will interest his patients in the care of the human frame, in diet and the cause and prevention of disease. – Thomas Edison, Inventor of the Electric light bulb and the phonograph

Avoid These Processed, Refined, Harmful Foods

Once you realize the harm caused to your body by unhealthy refined, chemicalized, deficient foods, you'll want to eliminate these "killer" foods. Also avoid microwaved foods! Follow The Bragg Healthy Lifestyle to provide the basic, healthy nourishment to maintain your health.

- Refined sugar, artificial sweeteners (toxic aspartame, Splenda) & their products as jams, jellies, preserves, marmalades, yogurts, ice cream, sherbets, Jello, cake, candy, cookies, chewing gum, colas & diet drinks, pies, pastries, and all sugared fruit juices and fruits canned in sugar syrup. **(Health Stores have delicious healthy replacements, Stevia, etc, so seek and buy the best. Page 101)**

- White flour products such as white bread, wheat-white bread, enriched flours, rye bread that has white flour in it, dumplings, biscuits, buns, gravy, pasta, pancakes, waffles, soda crackers, pizza, ravioli, pies, pastries, cakes, cookies, prepared and commercial puddings and ready-mix bakery products. Most made with dangerous (oxy-cholesterol) powdered milk and powdered eggs. **(Health Stores have huge variety of 100% whole grain organic products, delicious breads, crackers, pastas, desserts, etc.)**

- Salted foods, such as corn chips, potato chips, pretzels, crackers and nuts.

- Refined white rices and pearled barley. • Fast fried foods. • Indian ghee.

- Refined, sugared (also, aspartame), dry processed cereals – cornflakes etc.

 • Foods that contain olestra, palm and cottonseed oil. These additives are not fit for human consumption and should be totally avoided.

- Peanuts and peanut butter that contain hydrogenated, hardened oils and any peanut mold and all molds that can cause allergies.

- Margarine – combines heart-deadly trans-fatty acids and saturated fats.

- Saturated fats and hydrogenated oils – enemies that clog the arteries.

- Coffee, decaffeinated coffee, caffeinated green & caffeinated black tea. Also alcoholic beverages, caffeinated & sugared water-juices, cola & soft drinks.

- Fresh pork and products. • Fried, fatty greasy meats. • Irradiated GMO foods.

- Smoked meats, such as ham, bacon, sausage and smoked fish.

- Luncheon meats, hot dogs, salami, bologna, corned beef, pastrami and packaged meats containing dangerous sodium nitrate or nitrite.

- Dried fruits containing sulphur dioxide – a toxic preservative

- Don't eat chickens or turkeys that have been injected with hormones or fed with commercial poultry feed containing any drugs or toxins.

- Canned soups - read labels for sugar, salt, starch, flour and preservatives

- Foods containing benzoate of soda, salt, sugar, cream of tartar and any additives, drugs, preservatives; irradiated and genetically engineered foods.

- Day-old cooked vegetables, potatoes and pre-mixed, wilted lifeless salads.

- All commercial vinegars: pasteurized, filtered, distilled, white, malt and synthetic vinegars are the dead vinegars! *(We use only our Bragg Organic Raw, unfiltered Apple Cider Vinegar with "mother" as used in olden times.)*

HEALTHY HEART HABITS FOR A LONG, VITAL LIFE

Remember, *organic live foods make live people. You are what you eat, drink, breathe, think, say and do.* So eat a low-fat, low-sugar, high-fiber diet of organic whole grains, fresh salads, sprouts, greens, vegetables, fruits, raw seeds, nuts, fresh juices and chemical-free, purified or distilled water.

Earn your food with daily exercise, for regular exercise, power walking, etc. improves your health, stamina, go-power, flexibility, endurance and helps open the cardiovascular system. Only 45 minutes a day truly can do miracles for your heart, arteries, mind, nerves, soul and body! You become revitalized with new zest for living to accomplish your life goals!

We are made of tubes. To help keep them open, clean and to maintain good elimination, add 1 tsp psyllium husk powder or oat bran daily – hour after dinner to juices, herbal teas, even Bragg Vinegar Drink. Another way to guard against clogged tubes daily is to add 1-2 tsps soy lecithin granules (*fat emulsifier-melts like butter*) over potatoes, veggies, soups and to juices, etc. Also take one cayenne capsule (40,000 HU) daily with a meal. Take 50 to 100 mgs regular-released niacin (B-3) with one meal daily to help cleanse and open the cardiovascular system, also improves memory. Skin flushing may occur, don't worry about this as it shows it's working! After cholesterol level reaches 180, then only take niacin twice weekly.

The heart needs healthy balanced nutrients, so take natural multi-vitamin-mineral food supplements, Omega-3 and extra heart helpers – mixed vitamin E, C, CoQ10, MSM, D-Ribose, garlic, turmeric, selenium, zinc, beta carotene and amino acids, L-Carnitine, L-Taurine, L-Lysine and Proline. Folic acid, CoQ10, B6 and B12 helps keep homocysteine level low. Magnesium Orotate, Hawthorn Berry Extract brings relief for palpitations, arrhythmia, senile hearts and coronary disease. Braggzyme contains systemic enzymes (nattokinase and serrapetase) to keep blood thin, preventing dangerous blood clots. Take bromelain (from pineapple) also found in Braggzyme, multi-digestive enzyme and probiotics with meals – aids digestion, assimilation and elimination.

For sleep problems try 5-HTP Tryptophan (an amino acid), melatonin, calcium, magnesium, valerian in caps, extract or tea, Bragg vinegar drink and sleepytime herb tea. For arthritis or joint pain/stiffness, try aloe juice or gel, Braggzyme, Glucosamine - Chondroitin - MSM combo caps and shots, help heal and regenerate. Capsaicin and DMSO lotion helps relieve pain.

Use amazing antioxidants – natural vitamin mixed E, C, Quercetin, grapeseed extract (OPCs), CoQ10, selenium, SOD, Resveratrol, Alpha-Lipoic Acid, etc. They improve immune system and help flush out dangerous free radicals that cause havoc with cardiovascular pipes and health. Research shows antioxidants promote longevity, slows ageing, fights toxins, helps prevent disease, cancer, cataracts, jet lag and exhaustion.

Recommended Blood Chemistry Values

- **Diabetic Risk Tests:** • **Glucose:** 80-100 mg/dl • **HemoglobinA1c:** 7% or less
- **Homocysteine:** 6-8 μmol/L
- **CRP (C-reactive protein high sensitivity):**
    lower than 1 mg/L low risk, 1-3 mg/L average risk, over 3 mg/L high risk
- **Total Cholesterol:** Adults: 180 mg/dl is optimal; **Children:** 140 mg/dl or less
- **HDL Cholesterol:** Men: 50 mg/dl or more; **Women:** 65 mg/dl or more
- **HDL Cholesterol Ratio:** 3.2 or less • **Triglycerides:** 100 mg/dl or less
- **LDL Cholesterol:** 100 mg/dl or less is optimal
- **Blood Pressure:** 120/70 mmHg is considered optimal for adults

Iron Pumping Oldsters (86 to 96) Triple Their Muscle Strength in U.S. Study

WASHINGTON – Ageing nursing home residents in Boston study "pumping iron"? Elderly weightlifters tripling and quadrupling their muscle strength? Is it possible? Most people would doubt it! But government experts on ageing answered those questions with a resounding "yes" thanks to the results of this amazing landmark study! Visit web: *jcaaa.org/liftingweights.htm*

They turned a group of frail Boston nursing home residents, aged 86 to 96, into weightlifters to demonstrate that it's never too late to reverse age-related decline in muscle strength. The group participated in a regimen of high-intensity weight-training in a study conducted by Dr. Maria A. Fiatarone at Tufts University in Boston.

Amazing Strength Results in 8 Weeks

"The favorable response to strength training in our subjects was remarkable in light of their advanced ages and sedentary habits. The elderly weight-lifters increased their muscle strength by three-fold to four-fold in as little as eight weeks." Fiatarone said they were stronger at the end of the program than they had been in years! The results were amazing! Fiatarone emphasized the safety of such a closely supervised weight-lifting program, even among people in frail health. The average age of the participants was 90. Six had coronary heart disease; seven had arthritis; six had bone fractures resulting from osteoporosis; four had high blood pressure; and all had been physically inactive for years. Yet, no serious medical problems resulted from the strength exercise program. A few of the participants did report minor muscle and joint aches.

The study participants, faithfully worked out 3 times a week with hand weights and weight-lifting machines. The weights were gradually increased from 10 pounds to about 40 pounds at the end of the eight week program. Fiatarone said the study carries important health implications to improve the wellness and fitness of older people, who represent a growing proportion of the U.S. population. A decline in muscle strength, tone and muscle size is the more predictable feature of ageing.

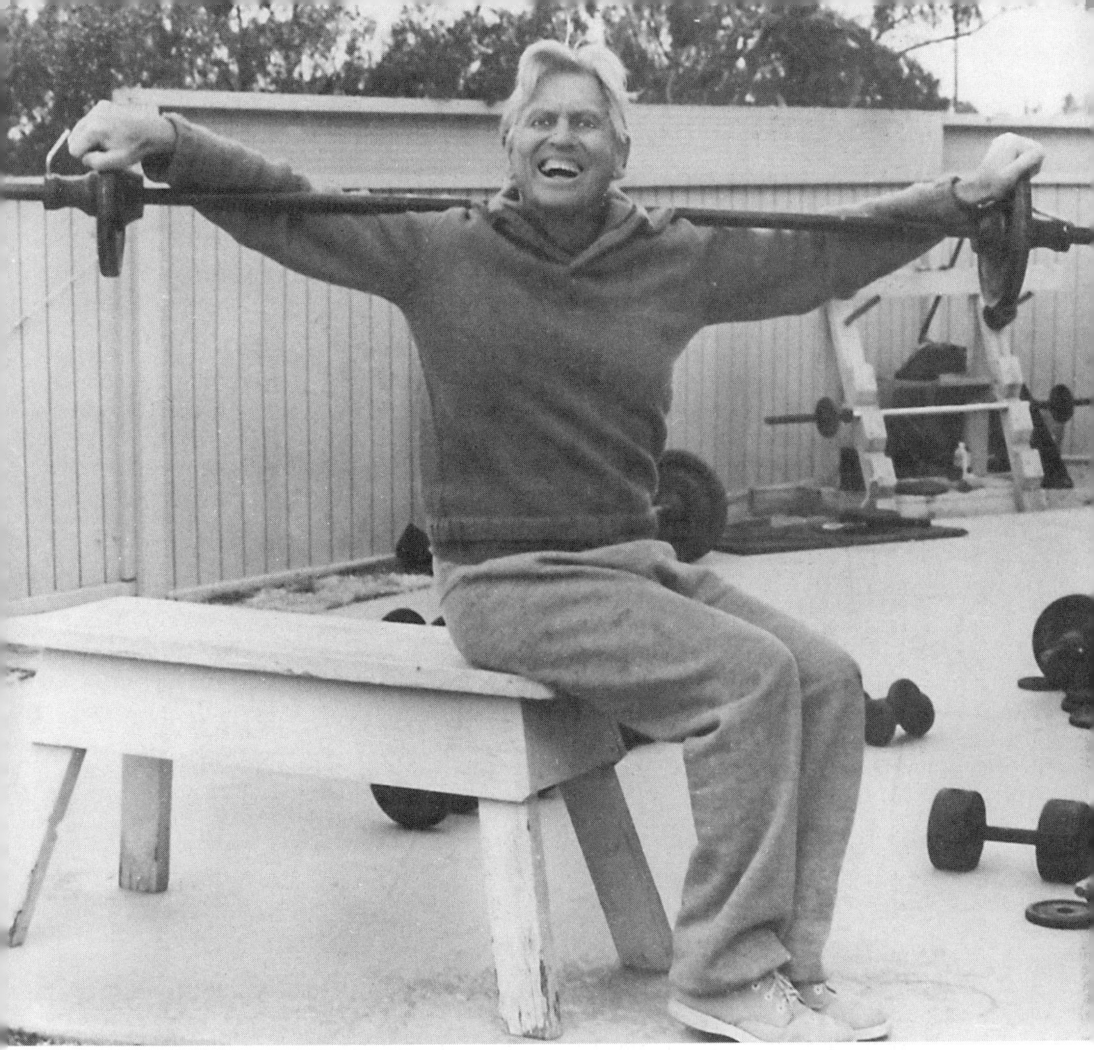

Paul C. Bragg and Patricia Lift Weights 3 Times Weekly

Building Up a Healthy Body with Exercise

Exercise helps to normalize blood pressure and create a healthy pulse. It keeps the blood flowing smoothly and not clot. Staying active keeps you feeling energized! Brisk walking is the best all-around exercise. Vow to become a health walker daily. Along with walking, we like to encourage you to use free-weights or dumbbells to build up your muscles. Lifting weights is a great compliment to the workout your legs get from walking. Keep your weights in the living room and use them as you watch TV in the evening. Even people well into their 70's, 80's and even 90's can be weight lifters. All you have to do is start. You'll never regret it.

Staying active is like riding an UP elevator. The more you do, the more you feel like staying involved. Even couch potatoes can become active and fit!

Fitness Promotes Health and Longevity
It's Never Too Late to Start!

Muscle strength in the average adult decreases by 30% to 50% during the course of life, mostly consequences of a sedentary unhealthy lifestyle and other controllable factors (*diet habits, etc.*). Muscle atrophy and weakness are not merely cosmetic problems with the frail elderly. Researchers now link muscle weakness with recurrent falls, a major cause of immobility and death in the American elderly population. This is causing millions of dollars yearly in staggering medical costs! Previous studies have also suggested weight-training can be helpful in reversing age-related muscle weakness. But Fiatarone said physicians have been reluctant to recommend weight-lifting for the frail elderly with multiple health problems. This new government study might be changing their minds! Also, this study shows great importance of keeping the 640 muscles as active and fit as possible to maintain general good health (page 73). Pioneer fitness crusader Dr. Kenneth Cooper of Dallas, Texas is dedicated to improving American's health, fitness and longevity. See his web: *www.cooperinst.org*.

90

Nature's Miracle Phytochemicals Help Prevent Cancer

Make sure to get your daily dose of these naturally occurring, cancer fighting biological substances, that are abundant in apples, onions, garlic, beans, legumes, soybeans, cabbage, cauliflower, broccoli, citrus fruits, etc. The winner tomatoes, which contains about 10,000 different phytochemicals!

Nutrition directly affects growth, development, reproduction, well-being of an individual's physical and mental condition. Health depends upon nutrition more than on any other single factor. – Dr. Wm. H. Sebrell, Jr.

Healthy Alternative Therapies and Massage Techniques

Try Them – They Work Miracles!

Explore these wonderful natural methods of healing your body. Finally over 600 Medical Schools in the U.S. are teaching Healthy Alternative Therapies. Now choose the best healing techniques for you:

ACUPUNCTURE/ACUPRESSURE Acupuncture directs and rechannels body energy by inserting hair-thin needles (*use only disposable needles*) at specific points on the body. It's used for pain, backaches, migraines and general health and body dysfunctions. Used in Asia for centuries, acupuncture is safe, virtually painless and has no side effects. **Acupressure** is based on the same principles and uses finger pressure and massage rather than needles. Websites offer info, check them out. Web: *acupuncturetoday.com*

CHIROPRACTIC Chiropractic was founded in Davenport, Iowa in 1885 by Daniel David Palmer. There are now many schools in the U.S., and graduates are joining Health Practitioners in all nations of the world to share healing techniques. Chiropractic is popular, is the largest U.S. healing profession benefitting literally millions. Treatment involves soft tissue, spinal and body adjustment to free the nervous system of interferences with normal body function. Its concern is the functional integrity of the musculoskeletal system. In addition to manual methods, chiropractors use physical therapy modalities exercise, health and nutritional guidance. Web: *chiroweb.com*

F. MATHIUS ALEXANDER TECHNIQUE These lessons help end improper use of neuromuscular system and bring body posture back into balance. Eliminates psycho-physical interferences, helps release long-held tension, and aids in re-establishing muscle tone. Web: *alexandertechnique.com*

FELDENKRAIS METHOD Dr. Moshe Feldenkrais founded this in the late 1940s. Lessons lead to improved posture and help create ease and efficiency of movement. This method is a great stress removal. Web: *feldenkrais.com*

91

Touch is a primal need and is as necessary for growth as food, clothing or shelter. Michelangelo knew this when he painted God extending a hand to Adam on the Sistine Chapel ceiling, he chose touch to depict the gift of life. – George H. Colt

Alternative Health Therapies & Massage Techniques

HOMEOPATHY In the 1800's, Dr. Samuel Hahnemann developed homeopathy. Patients are treated with minute amounts of substances similar to those that cause a particular disease to trigger the body's own defenses. The homeopathic principle is *Like Cures Like.* This safe and nontoxic remedy is the #1 alternative therapy in Europe and Britain because it is inexpensive, seldom has any side effects, and brings fast results. Web: *homeopathic.org*

NATUROPATHY Brought to America by Dr. Benedict Lust, M.D., this treatment uses diet, herbs, homeopathy, fasting, exercise, hydrotherapy, manipulation and sunlight. (Dr. Paul C. Bragg graduated from Dr. Lust's first School of Naturopathy in the U.S. Now 6 schools) Practitioners work with your body to restore health naturally. They reject surgery and drugs except as a last resort. Web: *naturopathic.org*

OSTEOPATHY The first School of Osteopathy was founded in 1892 by Dr. Andrew Taylor Still, M.D. There are now 15 U.S. colleges. Treatment involves soft tissue, spinal and body adjustments that free the nervous system from interferences that can cause illness. Healing by adjustment also includes good nutrition, physical therapies, proper breathing and good posture. Dr. Still's premise: if the body structure is altered or abnormal, then proper body function is altered and can cause pain and illness. Web: *osteopathic.org*

92

REFLEXOLOGY OR ZONE THERAPY Founded by Eunice Ingham, author of *Stories The Feet Can Tell*, inspired by a Bragg Health Crusade when she was 17. Reflexology helps the body by removing crystalline deposits from reflex areas (nerve endings) of feet and hands through deep pressure massage. Primative reflexology originated in China and Egypt and Native American Indians and Kenyans practiced it for centuries. Reflexology activates the body's flow of healing and energy by dislodging deposits. Visit Eunice Ingham and nephew Dwight Byer's web: *www.reflexology-usa.net*

SKIN BRUSHING daily is wonderful for circulation, toning, cleansing and healing. Use a dry vegetable brush (never nylon) and brush lightly. Helps purify lymph so it's able to detoxify your blood and tissues. Removes old skin cells, uric acid crystals and toxic wastes that come up through skin's pores. Use loofah sponge for variety in shower or tub.

Alternative Health Therapies & Massage Techniques

REIKI A Japanese form of massage that means "Universal Life Energy." Reiki helps the body to detoxify, then re-balance and heal itself. Discovered in the ancient Sutra manuscripts by Dr. Mikso Usui in 1822. Web: *reiki.org*

ROLFING Developed by Ida Rolf in the 1930's in the U.S. Rolfing is also called structural processing and postural release, or structural dynamics. It is based on the concept that distortions (accidents, injuries, falls, etc.) and the effects of gravity on the body cause upsets and long-term stress in the body. Rolfing helps to achieve balance and improved body posture. Methods involve the use of stretching, deep tissue massage, and relaxation techniques to loosen old injuries and break bad movement and posture patterns. Web: *rolf.org*

TRAGERING Founded by Dr. Milton Trager M.D., who was inspired at age 18 by Paul C. Bragg to become a doctor. It is a mind-body learning method that involves gentle shaking and rocking, allowing the body to let go, releasing tensions and lengthening the muscles for more body peace and health. Tragering can do miraculous healing where needed in the muscles and the entire body. Web: *trager.com*

WATER THERAPY Soothing detox shower: apply olive oil to skin, alternate hot and cold water, every 2-3 minutes. Massage body while under hot, filtered spray. Garden hose massage is great in summer or anytime. Hot detox soak bath (diabetics use warm water) 20 minutes with cup of Epsom salts or apple cider vinegar. This soak helps pull out the toxins by creating an artificial fever cleanse. Web: *holisticonline.com/hydrotherapy.htm*

MASSAGE & AROMATHERAPY works two ways: the essence (aroma) relaxes, as does the massage. Essential oils are extracted from flowers, leaves, roots, seeds and barks. These are usually massaged into the skin, inhaled or used in a bath for their ability to relax, soothe and heal. The oils, used for centuries to treat numerous ailments, are revitalizing and energizing for the body and mind. Example: Tiger balm, MSM, echinacea and arnica help relieve muscle aches. Avoid skin creams and lotions with mineral oil – it clogs the skin's pores. Use these natural oils for the skin: almond, apricot kernel, avocado, and I use Bragg Organic Olive Oil and mix with aromatic essential oils: rosemary, lavender, rose, jasmine, sandalwood, lemon-balm, etc. – 6 oz. oil and 6 drops of an essential oil. Web: *naha.org*

Alternative Health Therapies & Massage Techniques

MASSAGE – SELF Paul C. Bragg often said, "You can be your own best massage therapist, even if you have only one good hand." Near-miraculous health improvements have been achieved by victims of accidents or strokes in bringing life back to afflicted parts of their own bodies by self-massage and even vibrators. Treatments can be day or night, almost continual. Self-massage also helps achieve relaxation at day's end. Families and friends can learn and exchange massages; it's a wonderful sharing experience. Remember, babies love and thrive with daily massages, start from birth. Family pets also love soothing, healing touch of massages. Web: *coolnurse.com/massage.htm*

MASSAGE – SHIATSU Japanese form of health massage that applies pressure from the fingers, hands, elbows and even knees along the same points as acupuncture. Shiatsu has been used in Asia for centuries to relieve pain, common ills, muscle stress and to aid lymphatic circulation. Web: *shiatsu.org*

MASSAGE – SPORTS An important health support system for professional and amateur athletes. Sports massage improves circulation and mobility to injured tissue, enables athletes to recover more rapidly from myofascial injury, reduces muscle soreness and chronic strain patterns. Soft tissues are freed of trigger points and adhesions, thus contributing to improvement of peak neuro-muscular functioning and athletic performance.

MASSAGE – SWEDISH One of the oldest and the most popular and widely used massage techniques. This deep body massage soothes and promotes circulation and is a great way to loosen and relax tight muscles before and after exercise. Web: *massageden.com/swedish-massage.shtml*

Author's Comment: We have personally sampled many of these Alternative Therapies. It's estimated that soon America's health care costs will leap over $2 trillion. It's more important than ever to be responsible for our own health! This includes seeking holistic health practitioners who are dedicated to keeping us well by inspiring us to practice prevention! These Alternative Healing Therapies are also popular and getting results: aroma, Ayurvedic, biofeedback, color, guided imagery, herbs, music, meditation, magnets, saunas, tai chi, chi gong, Pilates, Rebounder, yoga, etc. Explore them and be open to improving your earthly temple for a healthy, happier, longer life. *Seek and find the best for your body, mind and soul.* – Patricia Bragg

Dr. John Westerdahl Is A Young Dedicated Health Crusader

John Westerdahl is a young dedicated true Health Crusader. He has spread the message of health throughout Hawaii via his radio talk show "Nutrition and You," and with his lectures and clinics on nutrition, weight control, stop-smoking, stop drugs and his HEARTBEAT Program, which promoted cardiovascular fitness. John's outreach especially in Hawaii has improved the health of thousands. He now continues to reach millions worldwide with the Bragg Health Crusades. See and hear his lecturers, etc. on *www.bragghealthinstitute.org*

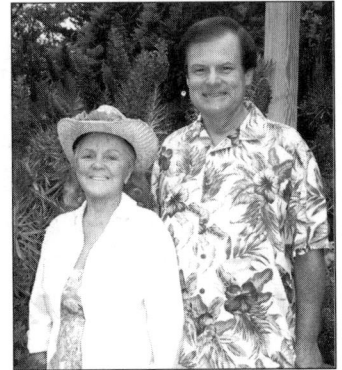

Dr. John was chosen as one of ten most outstanding young people of Hawaii. He justly deserved this high honor, for he's dedicated and loves being a Health Crusader! We at Health Science are proud of John and welcome him as the dynamic Director of the Bragg Health Institute. We encourage more young people into this Wellness Crusade to put America back where we belong, #1 in Health and Fitness instead of way down on the world list. – Patricia Bragg

Patricia Bragg with
Dr. John Westerdahl
Director of
Bragg Health Institute

The purest food is fruit, next vegetables, then the whole-grains. All pure poets have abstained almost entirely from animal food. Especially a minister should eat less meat, when he has to write and give a sermon. They say less meat, the better the sermon. – Louisa May Alcott

There is much false economy: those who are too poor to have the seasonable fruits and vegetables, will yet have pie and pickles all the year. They cannot afford oranges, yet can afford tea and coffee daily. – Health Calendar, 1910

If families could be induced to substitute the healthy organic apple, sound, ripe and luscious, in place of white sugar, white flour pies, cakes, candies and other sweets with which children are too often stuffed, then doctors' bills would diminish sufficiently enough in a year to pay for a whole season's eating pleasure of delicious, healthy apples.

DO MORE TO MAKE YOUR LIFE SUCCESSFUL

Do more than preach, practice.
Do more than think, ponder.
Do more than sympathize, empathize.
Do more than scold, set an example.
Do more than criticize, praise.
Do more than dream, make it a reality!
– *Rev. Paul Osumi, Honolulu, Hawaii*

HEALTHY BEVERAGES
Fresh Juices, Herb Teas & Energy Drinks

These freshly squeezed organic vegetable and fruit juices are important to The Bragg Healthy Lifestyle. It's not wise to drink beverages with your main meals, as it dilutes the digestive juices. But it's great during the day to have a glass of freshly squeezed orange, grapefruit, vegetable juice, Bragg Vinegar ACV Drink, herb tea or try hot cup Bragg Liquid Aminos Broth ($1/2$ to 1 tsp. Bragg Liquid Aminos in cup of hot distilled water) – these are all ideal pick-me-up beverages.

Bragg Apple Cider Vinegar Cocktail – Mix 1 to 2 tsps Bragg Organic ACV and (*optional*) to taste raw honey or pure maple syrup (*if diabetic, to sweeten use 2 Stevia herb drops or pinch of Stevia powder*) in 8 oz. of distilled or purified water. Take glass upon arising, hour before lunch and dinner.

Delicious Hot or Cold Cider Drink – Add 2 to 3 cinnamon sticks and 4 cloves to water and boil. Steep 20 minutes or more. Before serving add Bragg Vinegar and sweetener to taste (*Re-use cinnamon sticks & cloves*).

Bragg Favorite Juice Cocktail – This drink consists of all raw vegetables (please remember organic is best) which we prepare in our vegetable juicer: carrots, celery, beets, cabbage, tomatoes, watercress and parsley, etc. The great purifier, garlic we enjoy, but it's optional.

Bragg Favorite Healthy Energy Smoothie – After morning stretch and exercises we often enjoy this drink instead of fruit. It's delicious and powerfully nutritious as a meal anytime: lunch, dinner or take in thermos to work, school, sports, gym, hiking, and to park or freeze for popsicles.

96

Bragg Healthy Energy Smoothie

Prepare following in blender, add frozen juice cube if desired colder; Choice of: freshly squeezed orange or grapefruit juice; carrot and greens juice; unsweetened pineapple juice; or $1^1/2$ - 2 cups purified or distilled water with:

2 tsps spirulina or green powder
$1/3$ tsp Bragg Nutritional Yeast
2 dates or prunes, pitted (optional)
1 "Emergen-C" Vitamin C packet
1 tsp protein powder
$1/2$ tsp flax seed oil or 1 Tbsp seeds (grind)

1 to 2 bananas, ripe
   or fresh fruit in season
1-2 tsps almond or nut butter
$1/2$ tsp lecithin granules
1 tsp raw honey (optional)
$1/2$ tsp rice or oat bran

Optional: 4 apricots (sundried, unsulphured) soak in jar overnight in purified/distilled water or unsweetened pineapple juice. We soak enough to last for several days. Keep refrigerated. In summer you can add organic fresh fruit: peaches, papaya, blueberries, strawberries, all berries, apricots, etc. instead of banana. In winter, add apples, kiwi, oranges, tangelos, persimmons or pears, and if fresh is unavailable, try sugar-free, frozen organic fruits. Serves 1 to 2.

Patricia's Delicious Health Popcorn

Use freshly popped organic popcorn (use air popper). Try Bragg Organic Olive Oil or flax seed oil or melted salt-free butter over popcorn and add several sprays of Bragg Liquid Aminos and Bragg Apple Cider Vinegar – Yes, it's delicious! Now sprinkle with Bragg Nutritional Yeast Seasoning and Bragg Sprinkle (24 herbs & spices). For a variety try a pinch of cayenne pepper, mustard powder or fresh crushed garlic to oil mixture. Serve instead of breads!

Bragg Lentil & Brown Rice Casserole, Burgers or Soup
Jack LaLanne's Favorite Recipe

14 oz pkg lentils, uncooked
4 - 6 carrots, chop 1" rounds
3 celery stalks, chop, (optional)
2 onions, chop, (optional)
5-6 cups, distilled /purified water

1^1/2 cups brown organic rice, uncooked
4 garlic cloves, chop, (optional)
1 tsp Bragg Liquid Aminos
^{1}/4 tsp Bragg Sprinkle (24 Herbs & Spices)
2 tsps Bragg Organic Virgin Olive Oil

Wash & drain lentils & rice. Place grains in large stainless steel pot. Add water, bring to boil, reduce heat, then add vegetables & seasonings to grains and simmer for 30 minutes. If desired, last 5 minutes add fresh or canned (salt-free) tomatoes before serving. For delicious garnish add spray of Bragg Aminos, minced parsley & Bragg Nutritional Yeast Seasoning. Mash or blend for burgers. For soup, add more water. Serves 4 to 6.

Bragg Raw Organic Vegetable Health Salad

2 stalks celery, chop
1 bell pepper & seeds, dice
^{1}/2 cucumber, slice
2 carrots, grate
1 raw beet, grate
1 cup green cabbage, chop

^{1}/2 cup red cabbage, chop
^{1}/2 cup alfalfa or sunflower sprouts
2 spring onions & green tops, chop
1 turnip, grate
1 avocado (ripe)
3 tomatoes, medium size

For variety add organic raw zucchini, sugar peas, mushrooms, broccoli, cauliflower, (try black olives & pasta). Chop, slice or grate vegetables fine to medium for variety in size. Mix vegetables & serve on bed of lettuce, spinach, watercress or chopped cabbage. Dice avocado & tomato & serve on side as a dressing. Serve choice of fresh squeezed lemon, orange or dressing separately. Chill salad plates before serving. **It's best to always eat salad first before serving hot dishes.** Serves 3 to 5.

Bragg Health Salad Dressing

^{1}/2 cup Bragg Organic Apple Cider Vinegar
1-2 tsps organic raw honey

^{1}/2 tsp Bragg Liquid Aminos
1-2 cloves garlic, minced

^{1}/3 cup Bragg Organic Olive Oil, or blend with safflower, soy, sesame or flax oil
1 Tbsp fresh herbs, minced or pinch of Bragg Sprinkle (24 herbs & spices)

Blend ingredients in blender or jar. Refrigerate in covered jar.

FOR DELICIOUS HERBAL VINEGAR: In quart jar add ^{1}/3 cup tightly packed, crushed fresh sweet basil, tarragon, dill, oregano, or any fresh herbs desired, combined or singly. (If dried herbs, use 1-2 tsps. herbs.) Now cover to top with Bragg Organic Apple Cider Vinegar and store two weeks in warm place, and then strain and refrigerate.

Honey – Celery Seed Vinaigrette

^{1}/4 tsp dry mustard
^{1}/4 tsp Bragg Liquid Aminos
^{1}/4 tsp paprika or to taste
2-3 Tbsps raw honey or to taste

1 cup Bragg Organic Apple Cider Vinegar
^{1}/2 cup Bragg Organic Extra Virgin Olive Oil
^{1}/2 small onion, minced
^{1}/3 tsp celery seed (or vary amount to taste)

Blend ingredients in blender or jar. Refrigerate in covered jar.

Take Time for 12 Things

1. Take time to **Work** –
   it is the price of success.
2. Take time to **Think** –
   it is the source of power.
3. Take time to **Play** –
   it is the secret of youth.
4. Take time to **Read** –
   it is the foundation of knowledge.
5. Take time to **Worship** –
   it is the highway of reverence and
   washes the dust of earth from our eyes.
6. Take time to **Help and Enjoy Friends** –
   it is the source of happiness.
7. Take time to **Love and Share** –
   it is the one sacrament of life.
8. Take time to **Dream** –
   it hitches the soul to the stars.
9. Take time to **Laugh** –
   it is the singing that helps life's loads.
10. Take time for **Beauty** –
    it is everywhere in nature.
11. Take time for **Health** –
    it is the true wealth and treasure of life.
12. Take time to **Plan** –
    it is the secret of being able to have time
    for the first 11 things.

98

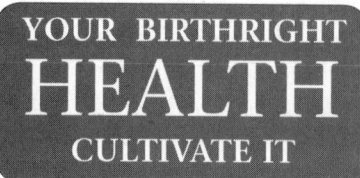

YOUR BIRTHRIGHT
HEALTH
CULTIVATE IT

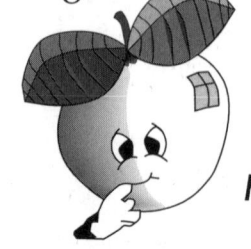

Have an
Apple
Healthy Life!

Teach me Thy way O Lord, and
lead me in a simple plain path. – Psalms 27:11

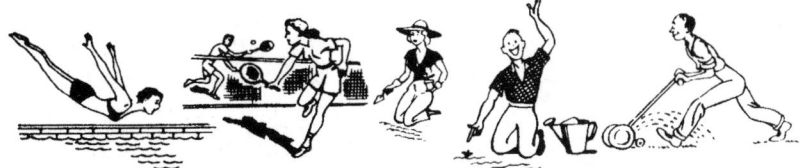

The Bragg Healthy Lifestyle
For a Lifetime of Super Health

In a broad sense, "The Bragg Healthy Lifestyle for the Total Person" is a combination of physical, mental, emotional, social and spiritual components. The ability of the individual to function effectively in his environment depends on how smoothly these components function as a whole. Of all the qualities that comprise an integrated personality, a totally healthy, fit body is one of the most desirable . . . so start today to achieve your health goals!

A person may be said to be totally physically fit if he functions as a total personality with efficiency and without pain or discomfort of any kind. This is to have a Painless, Tireless, Ageless Body, possessing sufficient muscular strength and endurance to maintain a healthy posture and successfully carry on the duties imposed by life and the environment, to meet emergencies satisfactorily and have enough energy for recreation and social obligations after the "work day" has ended. It is to meet the requirements of his environment through possessing the resilience to recover rapidly from fatigue, tension, stress and strain of daily living without the aid of stimulants, drugs or alcohol, and enjoy natural recharging sleep at night and awaken fit and alert in the morning for the challenges of the new fresh day ahead.

Keeping the body totally healthy and fit is not a job for the uninformed or the careless person. It requires an understanding of the body and of a healthy lifestyle and then following it for a long, happy lifetime of health! The result of "The Bragg Healthy Lifestyle" is to wake up the possibilities within you, rejuvenate your body, mind and soul to total balanced health. It's within your reach, so don't procrastinate, start today! Our hearts go out to touch your heart with nourishing, caring love for your total health, happiness and life!

Patricia Bragg and *Paul C. Bragg*

Dear friend, I wish above all things that thou may prosper and be in health even as the soul prospers. – 3 John 2

99

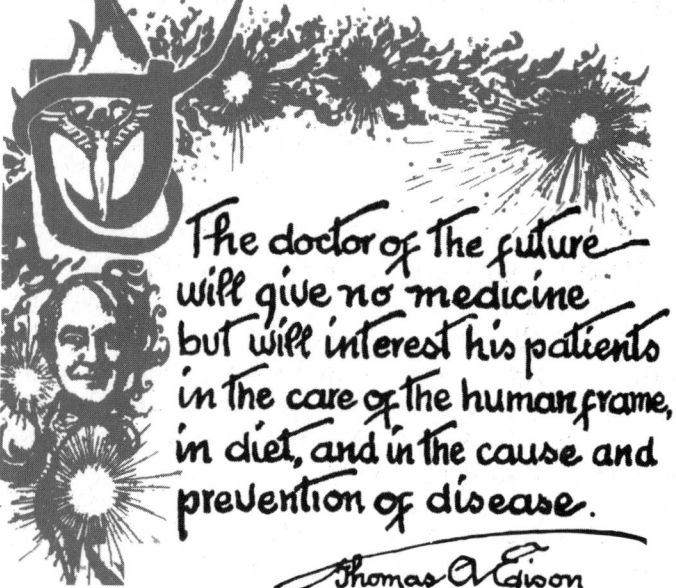

The doctor of the future will give no medicine but will interest his patients in the care of the human frame, in diet, and in the cause and prevention of disease.

— Thomas A. Edison

Eat More Healthy Fiber for Super Health

- EAT BERRIES, surprisingly good sources of fiber.

- KEEP BEANS HANDY, probably the best fiber sources. Cook dried beans and freeze in portions. Use canned beans for faster meals.

- INSTEAD OF ICEBERG LETTUCE, choose deep green lettuces (romaine, bib, butter, etc.), spinach or cabbage for variety salads.

- LOOK FOR "100% WHOLE WHEAT" or whole grain breads. A dark color isn't proof; check labels, compare fibers, grains, etc.

- WHOLE GRAIN CEREALS. Hot, also cold granolas with sliced fruit.

- GO FOR BROWN RICE. It's better for you and so delicious.

- EAT THE SKINS of potatoes and other fruits and vegetables.

- LOOK FOR CRACKERS with at least 2 grams of fiber per ounce.

- SERVE HUMUS, made from chickpeas, instead of sour-cream dips.

- USE WHOLE WHEAT FLOUR for baking breads, muffins, pastries, pancakes, waffles and for variety try other whole grain flours.

- DON'T UNDERESTIMATE CORN, including popcorn & corn tortillas.

- ADD OAT BRAN, WHEAT BRAN AND WHEATGERM to baked goods, cookies, etc.; whole grain cereals, casseroles, loafs, etc.

- SNACK ON SUN-DRIED FRUIT, such as apricots, dates, prunes, raisins, etc., which are concentrated sources of nutrients and fiber.

- INSTEAD OF DRINKING JUICE, eat the fruit: orange, grapefruit, etc.; and vegetables: tomato, carrot, etc. – *www.berkeleywellness.com*

Almost every known food may cause some allergic reaction at times. Thus, foods used in *elimination* diets may cause allergic reactions in some individuals. Some are listed among the *Most Common Food Allergies*. Since reaction to these foods is generally low, they are widely used in making test diets. By keeping a food journal and tracking your pulse rate after meals you will soon know your *problem* foods. Allergic foods cause pulse to go up. (Take base pulse before meals and then 30 minutes after meals. If it increases 8 -10 beats per minute – check foods for allergies.) See web: *www.vitaminlady.com/Articles/CocaPulseTest.asp*

If your body has a reaction after eating some particular food, especially if it happens each time you eat that food, you may have an allergy. Some allergic reactions are: wheezing, sneezing, stuffy nose, nasal drip or mucus, dark circles, eye watering or waterbags under eyes, headaches, feeling light-headed or dizzy, fast heart beat, stomach or chest pains, diarrhea, extreme thirst, breaking out in a rash, swelling of extremities or stomach bloating, etc. (Do read Dr. Arthur Coca's book, *The Pulse Test* – available: *amazon.com*)

If you know what you're allergic to, you are lucky; if you don't, you had better find out as fast as possible and eliminate all irritating foods from your diet. To re-evaluate your daily life and have a health guide to your future, start a daily journal (8 1/2 x 11 notebook pg.102) of foods eaten, your pulse rate after meals and your reactions, moods, energy levels (ups and downs), weight, elimination and sleep patterns. You will discover the foods and situations causing problems. By charting your diet you will be amazed at the effects of eating certain foods. We have kept daily journals for years.

If you are hypersensitive to certain foods, you must omit them from your diet! There are hundreds of allergies and of course it's impossible here to take up each one. Many have allergies to milk, wheat, or some are allergic to all grains. Visit web: *foodallergy.org*. Your daily journal will help you discover and accurately pinpoint the foods and situations causing you problems. Start your journal today!

Most Common Food Allergies

- *MILK: Butter, Cheese, Cottage Cheese, Ice Cream, Milk, Yogurt, etc.*
- *CEREALS & GRAINS: Wheat, Corn, Buckwheat, Oats, Rye*
- *EGGS: Cakes, Custards, Dressings, Mayonnaise, Noodles*
- *FISH: Shellfish, Crabs, Lobster, Shrimp, Shadroe*
- *MEATS: Bacon, Beef, Chicken, Pork, Sausage, Veal, Smoked Products*
- *FRUITS: Citrus Fruits, Melons, Strawberries*
- *NUTS: Peanuts, Pecans, Walnuts, chemically dried preserved nuts*
- *MISCELLANEOUS: Chocolate, Black Tea, Cocoa, Coffee, MSG, Palm and Cottonseed Oils, Salt, Spices and allergic reactions often caused by toxic pesticides on salad greens, vegetables, fruits, etc.*

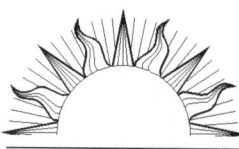

MY DAILY HEALTH JOURNAL

Today is:____/____/____

> **I have said my morning resolve and am ready to practice
> The Bragg Healthy Lifestyle today and every day.**

Yesterday I went to bed at: Today I arose at: Weight:

Today I practiced the No-Heavy Breakfast or No-Breakfast Plan: ☐ yes ☐ no

• For Breakfast I drank: Time:

  For Breakfast I ate: Time:

  Supplements:

• For Lunch I ate: Time:

  Supplements:

• For Dinner I ate: Time:

  Supplements:

• _____Glasses of Water I Drank during the Day

  List Snacks – Kind and When:

• **I took part in these physical (walking, gym, etc.) activities today:**

Grade each on scale of 1 to 10 (desired optimum health is 10).

• **I rate my day for the following categories:**

Previous Night's Sleep:	Stress/Anxiety:
Energy Level:	Elimination:
Physical Activity, Exercise:	Health:
Peacefulness:	Accomplishments:
Happiness:	Self-Esteem:

• **General Comments, Reactions and To Do List:**

Household Cleaning Hints with Vinegar

We don't endorse white vinegar or dead vinegars for human use – internally nor externally! But it seems well-suited for a variety of household and workshop chores. **White vinegar is an effective and inexpensive household cleaner, deodorizer and disinfectant;** which replaces commercial household cleaners that are full of chemicals and additives harmful to Mother Nature and you. But please remember: use only the healthiest – Bragg raw, organic unfiltered apple cider vinegar (*with "mother enzyme"*) for all human consumption and for your skin and hair.

VINEGAR USES FOR CLEANING KITCHEN AND FOODS*

• **Appliances and Countertops:** clean and disinfect with a white vinegar-dampened sponge or cloth.

• **Greasy Areas:** mix 1/4 cup white vinegar with 2 cups hot water and add 1 to 2 dashes of biodegradable liquid soap. (Keep mixture in handy, labeled spray bottle.)

• **Sponges and Dish Rags:** disinfect and deodorize by soaking overnight in 1 quart hot water with 1/4 cup vinegar.

• **Chopping and Bread Boards:** wipe down with full-strength white vinegar to disinfect - leave overnight; or sprinkle with baking soda before spraying with vinegar, wait an hour before wiping clean, then rinse with water.

• **Pots and Pans:** clean and polish with a paste of baking soda and white vinegar. Remove stubborn, stuck-on food with a 50/50 white vinegar-water soak.

• **Glass and China:** stop spotting by mixing 1/2 cup white vinegar in dishwater, or by placing 1 cup vinegar on bottom rack of electric dishwasher before starting wash.

• **Drains and Pipes:** keep fresh-smelling and free-flowing with 1/3 cup of baking soda followed by a cup of white vinegar. Cover drain opening with plate for an hour or longer before flushing through with cold water.

• **Garbage Disposals:** keep clean by grinding up frozen white vinegar ice cubes once weekly (80/20 vinegar-water solution to make cleansing ice cubes).

---

* *Wash vegetables, salad greens and fruits in a vinegar wash (1/3 cup white vinegar to 2–3 cups water) to help remove sprays, etc.* – Patricia Bragg

---

Remember, Cleanliness is next to Godliness.

• **Chrome and Stainless Steel**: straight white vinegar will disinfect and polish fixtures; apply with sponge, then buff with soft cloth.

• **Garbage Pails**: disinfect with a warm water and white vinegar solution. Let set for an hour or overnight.

• **Shower Curtains**: put through washer rinse cycle with 1 to 2 cups white vinegar. Spray occasionally with 50/50 vinegar-water solution to help prevent mold.

• **Sink, Tub and Shower**: spray with 80/20 vinegar-water mixture, leave 10 minutes, then scrub and rinse.

• **Toilet Bowl**: use 1/2 cup straight white vinegar, let stand an hour or overnight and flush. For bad stains, follow vinegar with biodegradable cleanser, after 2 hours brush and flush. If stains persist use Clorox bleach (1/2 cup) overnight.

VINEGAR USES FOR THE LAUNDRY ROOM

• **Washer Tub and Hoses:** remove soap accumulations by running machine for full cycle with pint of white vinegar.

• **New Clothes, Linens, etc:** to remove manufacturing chemicals and new smell odors, add 1 to 2 cups white vinegar to first wash before using. (Never use toxic perfume soaps.)

• **Perspiration Odors (clothes, socks, etc.) and Stained Clothes:** soak overnight in 1/4 cup vinegar and enough water to cover or soak in washer or pan, then wash in morning.

• **Clothes Final Rinse Cycle:** to help remove static and lint add 1/2 cup white vinegar.

• **To Soften and Disinfect Fabric, Clothes, Diapers, etc:** add 1/4 cup white vinegar to most laundry loads. (Don't ever use toxic fabric softeners – irritates skin.)

• **Fruit and Grass Stains:** dab with straight white vinegar best within 24 hours to safely remove most stains and spots.

• **Musky Smells:** to remove odor and freshen clean cotton clothes just sprinkle with white vinegar and press.

• **Steam Iron Plate:** to eliminate mineral deposits, fill iron reservoir with straight white vinegar and allow to steam on rag, then fill with plain water and turn upside down and let water drain out.

• **Scorched Fabric:** gently rub with white vinegar, then wipe with clean, white cloth.

VINEGAR USES FOR FLOORS, WALLS & FURNITURE

• **Floors:** sponge mop with 1 cup of white vinegar in a bucket of warm water. Also removes dull residue left by most commercial toxic cleaners.

• **Carpets:** light stains are extracted by using a mix of 2 Tbsps. salt and $1/2$ cup white vinegar, rub the paste mix into carpet and allow to dry before vacuuming.

• **Furniture:** remove cloudy look and brighten by rubbing with mixture of 1 Tbsp. vinegar in quart warm water, then buff with a soft cloth. Remove white rings and scratches from wood tables with a mix of 50/50 vinegar and olive oil or use only olive oil.

• **Vinyl Surfaces:** wipe down with 2 Tbsps. liquid soap and $1/2$ cup white vinegar, then water rinse and dry.

• **Toys:** Clean and disinfect with a light spray of vinegar (50/50 vinegar-water solution) and brush or wipe clean.

• **Air Freshener:** mask kitchen odors by simmering a pot of water with $1/2$ cup white vinegar.

• **Windows** (also shower doors): spray 50/50 vinegar-water mix, then wipe clean with squeegee. (Great for eye glasses.)

105

VINEGAR USES FOR OUTSIDE

• **Ants:** spray equal parts vinegar and water on areas where ant invasions start and surrounding areas. (Chili powder and salt also work.) Vinegar works as a non-toxic pesticide.

• **Car & Car Windows:** keep frost-free with coating solution of 50/50 white vinegar to water. Also, dissolve old decals and chewing gum with straight white vinegar.

• **Paint Brushes:** soften by soaking in boiling white vinegar; also, remember that vinegar absorbs paint odors!

• **Fresh-Cut Flowers:** to preserve add 2 tsps. vinegar to qt. warm water in vase. Cut ends & renew water every 3 days.

• **Unwanted Grass & Weeds:** pour on straight vinegar.

God will not change the condition of men,
until they change what is in themselves. – Koran

There is no such thing as too many friends, just as there is
never too much happiness! – Jean de La Bruyere

Never underestimate the power of a kind word or deed.

Happiness is a rainbow in your heart – a real health sparkler!
– Patricia Bragg, N.D., Ph.D., Health Crusader & Lifestyle Educator

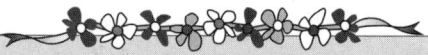

Our Favorite Quotes We Share with You . . .
where space allows. We all need inspiring, informative words of wisdom to help guide us in our daily living.

Here's a wise ancient Turkish saying: No matter how far you've gone down on a wrong road, turn back and get on the right road!

I cannot overstate the importance of the habit of quiet meditation and prayer for more health of body, mind and spirit. – Patricia Bragg

Breathing is the movement of spirit within the body; and working with breathing is a form of spiritual practice. – Andrew Weil, M.D.

Dream big, think big, but enjoy the small miracles of everyday life.

When you live The Bragg Healthy Lifestyle *you activate your own powerful internal defense arsenal and help maintain it at top efficiency.*

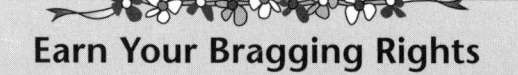

Earn Your Bragging Rights
Live The Bragg Healthy Lifestyle
To Attain Super Health & Enjoy Longevity

Health Crusaders Paul C. Bragg and daughter Patricia traveled the world spreading health, inspiring millions to renew and revitalize their health and life.

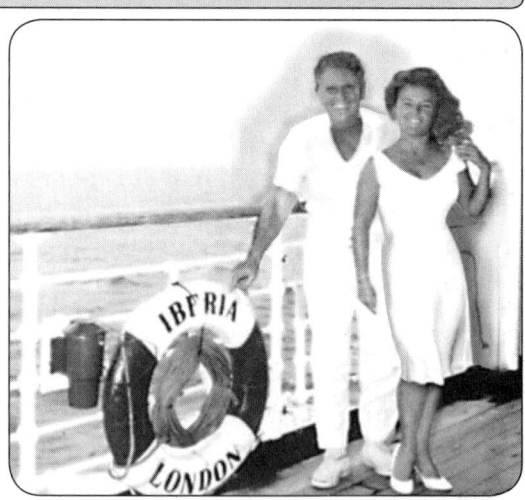

The Bragg books are written to inspire and guide you to health, fitness and longevity. Remember, the book you don't read won't help. So please read and reread the Bragg Books and live The Bragg Healthy Lifestyle!

With Blessings of Health, Peace, Joy and Love,

Paul and *Patricia*

We are recharged and blessed by each one of you reading our teachings. They are filled with health wisdom and love for you – thank you! – Patricia Bragg

Also follow Patricia and get Bragg Health Messages on twitter.com/patriciabragg

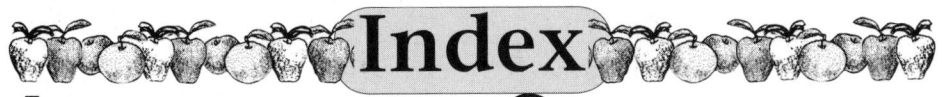

Index

A

Acid Crystals, 30, 33, 36, 40
Acne 25, 111, 115
Acupuncture/Acupressure, 91
Ageing, 5, 6, 33, 36, 40-41, 46, 70, 87
Alcohol 18, 43, 52, 59
Allergies 4, 18, 49, 101
Alternative Therapies 91-94
Amino Acids, 3, 7, 29-31, 57, 63, 87, 96-97
Animals 12-13, 34, 52, 55
Apple Cider Vinegar 1-4, 10-41, 50, 96
Apples 3, 5, 12, 49, 65, 95
Aromatherapy 93
Arrhythmia 27, 87
Arteries 5, 7, 12, 33, 38, 52, 67, 69, 73
Arthritis c, 15, 26, 30-31, 36, 40, 56, 84, 87
Asthma 21, 56, 70, 76
Athlete's Foot 25, 116

B

Bacteria 3
Baldness 26
Bee Stings, Bites 25, 111
Bedwetting 28
Beverages 31, 44, 63-67, 96 (recipes)
Biblical use of ACV 1
Bladder, problems dribbles 28, 70
Bleeding 32
Blood, Chemistry Values 87 (chart)
Blood Pressure 4, 27, 38, 115-116
Blood Sugar 44, 54, 57, 76
Bloodstream 5, 8, 38, 43-44, 83
Bowel Health b, 18, 29, 32-33, 47, 87
Bragg Healthy Recipes 96-97
Bragg Healthy Lifestyle xi, 11, 12,
    16-19, 28, 31, 33-34, 37-41,
    43-45, 55-56, 66, 73, 79, 99
Bragg, Paul iii, 9, 12-16, 35, 49-50, 106
Breakfast 50-51
Breathing 44, 48, 70, 75, 79, 106
Bronchitis 21
Burns 22, 24, 35
Bursitis 36

C

Cabbage 56, 97 (salad recipe)
Caffeine, (coffee) 4, 13, 18, 43, 50
Calcium 5, 12, 40, 67, 72 (chart), 87
Cancer d, 30, 54, 70, 84, 90
Cataracts 71, 87
Cells 7-8, 43-44, 46, 48, 70
Cellulite 16, 92
Children 11, 25, 33-34, 39, 47, 51, 87
Chiropractic 91
Cholesterol c, 4, 7, 12, 27, 41, 83, 87, 115
Chronic Fatigue 4, 13
Cleaning with vinegar 3, 103-105
Cocktail, ACV 11-12, 16-17, 28,
    30-32, 37-38, 41, 50
Colds 21, 24 (sores), 49, 111-112
Constipation b, 32-33, 47-48, 51, 79
CoQ10, 27, 38, 87
Corns & Callouses 20
Cramps 26, 40, 116
Cuts & Abrasions 24

D

Dairy Products 16, 18, 28, 31, 84, 86, 108
Dandruff 26
Deodorant 1
Depression, mental 5, 15, 45
Diabetes d, 11, 15, 112, 114, 117
Diaper Rash 25
Digestion 27-28, 33, 51, 55, 67, 87
Distilled Water 16-17, 19, 22,
    27-32, 38, 40, 66-71, 87
Douche 30

E

Ear Infections 25, 38
Eczema 25, 117
Elderly, pumping iron 88-90
Emphysema 21
Energy 7, 18, 22, 27, 45-46,
    48, 55, 58, 67-72, 115
Enzymes 3, 5, 13, 17, 29, 37, 87
Exercise iv, 9, 20, 68, 73-80, 83, 87-90, 110
Eyes 2, 5-6, 15, 18, 71 (eyewash), 115

"I conceive that a knowledge of books is the basis on which all other knowledge rests." – George Washington, 1st U.S. President

Kindness should be a frame of mind in which we are alert to every opportunity: to do, to give, to share and to cheer. – Patricia Bragg

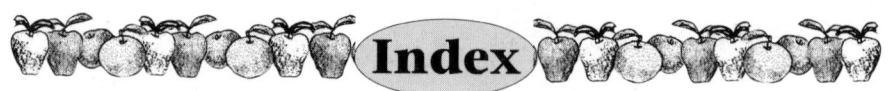

Index

Always do what is right – despite any public opinions.

What sunshine is to flowers, smiles are to humanity. – Joseph Addison

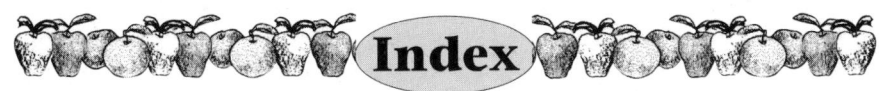

Index

Who you are speaks so loudly, I can't hear what you're saying.
– Ralph Waldo Emerson

*Love is not a matter of counting the years –
it's making the years count.* – William Smith

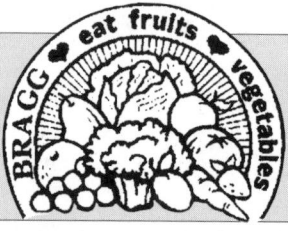

**GO ORGANIC!
DON'T PANIC!**

**GUARD YOUR
TOTAL HEALTH**

FROM THE AUTHORS

This book was written for You! It can be your passport to a healthy, long, vital life. We in the Alternative Health Therapies join hands in one common objective – promoting a high standard of health for everyone. Healthy nutrition points the way – which is Mother Nature and God's Way. This book teaches you how to work with them, not against them! Health Doctors, therapists nurses, teachers and caregivers are becoming more dedicated than ever before to keeping their patients healthy and fit. This book was written to emphasize the great needed importance of healthy lifestyle living for health and longevity, close to Mother Nature and God.

Statements in this book are scientific health findings, known facts of physiology and biological therapeutics. Paul C. Bragg practiced natural methods of living for over 80 years with highly beneficial results, knowing that they were safe and of great value. His daughter Patricia lectured and co-authored the Bragg Health Books with him and continues to carrying on The Bragg Health Crusades.

Paul C. Bragg and daughter Patricia express their opinions solely as Public Health Educators and Health Crusaders. They offer no cure for disease. Only the body has the ability to cure a person. Experts may disagree with some of the statements made in this book. However, such statements are considered to be factual, based on the long-time experience of dedicated pioneer health crusaders Paul C. Bragg and Patricia Bragg. If you suspect you have a medical problem, please always seek qualified health care professionals to help you make the healthiest, wisest and best-informed choices!

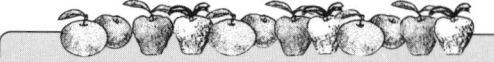

Count your blessings daily while you do your 30 to 45 minute brisk walks and exercises with these affirmations – health! strength! youth! vitality! peace! laughter! humility! understanding! forgiveness! joy! and love for eternity! – and soon all these qualities will come flooding and bouncing into your life. With blessings of super health, peace and love to you, our dear friends – our readers. – Patricia Bragg

If I were to name the three most precious resources of life, I would say books, friends and nature; and the greatest of these, at least the most constant and always at hand is Mother Nature and God. – John Burroughs

Peace is not a season, it is a way of life.

Change your mind and you change your life.

Praises for Apple Cider Vinegar & The Bragg Healthy Lifestyle

I was having 15 to 20 hot flashes a day and tried just about everything including homeopathy and acupuncture with no results. A week ago a friend told me about Bragg Apple Cider Vinegar for menopause discomforts so I tried it right away and what a gift from heaven! After a couple days of taking 3 to 4 vinegar drinks a day of the apple cider vinegar all my hot flashes are gone! This is too good to be true! Thank you for this miracle! – Maria Rodriguez, Capitola, CA

Having gone off HRT recently, hot flashes have been a real problem. Someone wrote into Dear Abby recently asking about a hot flash cure they had seen in the column. The formula was 2 tsps honey, 2 tsps apple cider vinegar in 8 oz of water 3 times a day (some need 2 Tbsps ACV). Sounded much too easy, but in no more than 3 days, the hot flashes had tapered off. I am now able to sleep at night. I've shared this with several friends and they have had the same amazing results! Thank you, it's been a miracle for sure. Thank you! – Jan Moore

I've been using Bragg's ACV for 5 years now and love the effects it has on my skin! It has also helped clear up acne and excessive oil issues. Now, I use ACV in my Holistic Health Practice where I council private clients in achieving a healthier lifestyle through easy improvements in their diet. ACV is something I include, free of charge with my program because I believe in it so thoroughly!
– Nancy Caballero, NY

I'm a big Paul Bragg fan and I also daily use Bragg Liquid Aminos on my food. I even take it with me when I travel for my seminars, I wouldn't be without it! The world and I are blessed with Bragg health teachings!
– Anthony "Tony" Robbins, www.anthony robbins.com

I just want to say how wonderful your apple cider vinegar is and what it has done for me and my family! First time I used it was when my son was allergic to mosquito bites. I gave him a compress soaked with your apple cider vinegar and it worked!!! Our whole family treats bites with it now. Any time my kids get colds or suffer from sinus we include this in our diet and have noticed a difference also. Thanks Bragg for your high quality health products! – Laura Bunderson, Glenwood, Iowa

My parents who are 91 and 86 are enjoying the Bragg ACV drink. I know it helps with so many things!!! I appreciate you and your kindness more than you know!!! – Barbara Magiley, San Antonio, TX

Praises for Apple Cider Vinegar & The Bragg Healthy Lifestyle

The pain in my right knee was unbearable. I bought the Bragg Vinegar Book. I took 2 tsp of ACV in 6 oz. water taken one hour before meals. It didn't take even a month to completely relieve my knee of all pain. I have passed on the word to all my friends. – C. Evelyn Sutcliffe, Clovis, CA

Thank you Patricia for our first meeting in London in 1968. You gave me your Fasting Book, it got me exercising, brisk walking and eating more wisely. You were a blessing God-sent. – Reverend Billy Graham

I bought and read *Miracle of Fasting* e-book twice (plan to read it many more times). I feel blessed to have found your website, e-books and the Bragg Health Lifestyle. Thank you so much. – Rick Cratty, Plymouth, MA

Your products are just great. I have been using Bragg Apple Cider Vinegar and Liquid Aminos for years. I would never consider using soy sauce ever again! I use Bragg's in cooking all the time. Thanks for great health products. Keep up the Health Crusading. – Glenda Berkley, Brockton, MA

Rock and roll health is better than rock and roll wealth. Thanks to Bragg, the road ain't a drag anymore! We thank Bragg for the super smooth going and success on our recent successful whirlwind 20 city tour of England. – David Polemeni, Boy's Town Band, Fort Lee, NJ

I love the Bragg All Natural Ginger & Sesame Salad Dressing that I bought here in Louisiana. It's so delicious! Also I am now enjoying all your health products! I regained my health by eating organic foods and vegetables and taking natural supplements. I'm eating foods the way God created them and my body is thriving. Thanks for your healthy delicious salad dressings. – Candace Hawthorne, Metairie, LA

I especially like your Bragg Aminos. My mother uses it in her recipes. – Mary Pierce, Former French Open Tennis Champion

I was diagnosed with diabetes and had high sugar levels. Within 6 months, I was insulin free! I am healthier now than I have been for the last 15 years. My wife, three young children and I are now all vegetarians and living the Bragg Healthy Lifestyle. The results have been amazing! We all thank You. – Dennis Urbans, Australia

Praises for Apple Cider Vinegar & The Bragg Healthy Lifestyle

In the past our family has had chronic health problems. Within the last year and a half God has shown us His Will for healing and divine health. Our journey has included a healthy diet, some fasting and a complete change in lifestyle. We tried ACV and I want you to know that it is one of the most valuable changes that we have included in our lifestyle! It is terrific! I cannot express how good we feel! I am so thankful for every good thing that God has put before us – this journey, and every miraculous result and ACV is part of that. Thank you for sharing this wealth of health in Bragg Books. God Bless You! – Rhonda Jackson, Blair, OK

Our lives have completely turned around all because of Bragg! Our family is feeling so very healthy and good, we must tell you about it.
– Gene & Joan Zollner, Parents of 11, Bellingham, WA

In my youth, (working around toxic asbestos) I inhaled asbestos fibers which the doctors told me there is no way to clean it out and no cure. I was not feeling well and my chest hurt. A friend of mine introduced me to Bragg Organic Apple Cider Vinegar Cocktail. I drink it 3 times a day and use it over my salads and veggies. I now feel very healthy and strong! What a blessing. I thank you for such a great product and your vinegar book on all the ways to use apple cider vinegar. I will continue to follow your teachings. Thank You. – Al Escalera, Santa Barbara, CA

I read your book on Bragg Organic Apple Cider Vinegar and now I take it daily. After passing the book on to my mom, she started using it and the pain in her shoulder that had been waking her up for years has vanished! We both thank you. – Catherine Cox, Toronto, Canada

---

The results with Bragg Vinegar and lifestyle are miraculous! I got rid of a constant cold and mucus. I feel so good, energetic and healthy again. Thank You! – Nestor R. Villagra, Toronto, Ontario, Canada

---

It was in Hawaii I began to realize that while lifestyle choices can not only be a major negative to health and well-being, but lifestyle can be a winning asset to wellness! My discovery on fitness and health began shortly after I arrived in Hawaii at 19 when I discovered fitness and health pioneer Paul Bragg teaching a free exercise class 6 days a week at Waikiki Beach.
– Kathy Smith, Hollywood, CA (www.kathysmith.com)

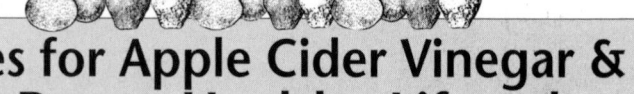

Praises for Apple Cider Vinegar & The Bragg Healthy Lifestyle

Several years ago a Physicians Assistant told me that a good way to avoid viruses was to take a Tbsp of Organic Raw Apple Cider Vinegar daily, mixed into water. He claimed that a virus couldn't survive an acidic environment. I began using that prevention method and I can't even remember the last time I had a cold or virus. Thanks for such a great useful health product! – Mike Freeman, Ekalaka, MT

I just tried your Apple Cider Vinegar. It is the BEST I have ever had. Recently, I went to a new doctor, Internal & Alternative Medicine. Taking your products has made my taste buds sing. Thanks for helping me find a healthy and happy energetic new me! Looking forward to enjoying more of your healthy products. – Jane Prestup, East Brunswick, NJ

Your ACV book saved me from having my gallbladder out. It's been 3-4 years since I started your Apple Cider Vinegar drink and it worked along with some healing prayers at church! I swear by it and think all Health and Book Stores should carry your book. I am grateful you wrote it. God Bless You. – Carmen Puro, Traverse City, MI

I was a diabetic and my blood sugar has been way out of whack for about a year, routinely hitting 300+. I was desperate and read about your Apple Cider Vinegar. I tried it and have been using it twice a day for a month – once in the morning and once in the evening – a shot of it in a glass of cold filtered water, no honey (would that even mix in cold water?) but here's the point – my blood sugar is now normal, rarely over 110 and I swear I have changed absolutely nothing else in my diet, exercise or medication. I am double checking it by using two different meters and different test strip lots, etc. I am astounded, amazed and just find it hard to believe it's possible! But it sure seems to be for real!!! Thanks!– Don Hess, Quincy, IL

I have just recently embraced the live food diet and I am so overwhelmed at the beauty and simplicity of it all. When we become aligned with Natural Laws the Universe opens up for you and nature does reveal it's mysteries to you! Apple Cider Vinegar is so much more than I ever realized. I am now drinking your ACV drink 3 times daily. It is like food of the gods. It is so nourishing. I bathe in it, rinse my hair in it, gargle with it and wash my clothes in it. I have eliminated most all of the totally toxic soaps, shampoos, cleansers and detergents from my home. What an amazing product ACV is!!! I love it and just want everyone to feel as good as I do!!! – Patrick McLean, Scammon, KS

Praises for Apple Cider Vinegar & The Bragg Healthy Lifestyle

I cannot say enough about this amazing product. It is just too good. I have been using it for almost 4 years and have lost about 80 lbs. I've bought and shared your Apple Cider Vinegar with family and friends who want to lose weight, cut their cholesterol, high blood pressure, sore throat, indigestion and so on. This product is extremely beneficial. What's there to lose? A whole lot of bad stuff. I tell them get started – it works miracles! – Anil Dutt, Sacramento, CA

After using your Apple Cider Vinegar & Honey mix for two weeks along with health ideas expressed in your *Apple Cider Vinegar* Book, I have noticed remarkable improvement in my joints. It is almost unbelievable how fast this has helped! Thanks. – Tyrone Robinson, St. Louis, MO

My husband suffered from gout for several years. He is a healthy, in-shape, 42 year old man. No one could figure out why he had gout in the first place, never mind trying to figure out how to treat it. The doctors prescribed him every medication you could possibly imagine. Nothing helped, in fact I think they made the problem worse. Just by chance a co-worker mentioned Bragg Apple Cider Vinegar. My husband went from being almost crippled, to not having a flare up in a year (ever since he started drinking the ACV drink). All I can do is thank you. Your product has saved him from a lifetime of chronic, excruciating pain. You cannot put a price on the quality of life. – Sue Stearnes, San Diego, CA

I just read my first Bragg book the *Apple Cider Vinegar Miracle Health System*. I am a believer!! I will be looking for the rest of your books. It is the most uplifting, honest, easy to read, informative book ever on health, nutrition and a positive mind, thank you. – Robyn Scollo, Rochester, NY

Thank you for existing! This is the best product that I have tried and felt the need to say it to you. Just finished eating the chopped Cabbage Salad which would be nothing without mighty Apple Cider Vinegar!! Thank You! – Dragan Petrovic, Israel

I use your Organic Apple Cider Vinegar for leg cramps. Also ACV is the ONLY thing I have found in 15 years that calmed my restless-leg-syndrome. Thanks so much! – Audra Lynn Weathers, Woodruff, SC

I LOVE Bragg Apple Cider Vinegar! My mom and I both drink it as shots straight up! It cures heartburn and indigestion I've had since gallbladder surgery. I also found that it works wonders for athletes foot and also takes off warts! Works for everything! Plus I just love the taste! Keep up the great work, I will always use Bragg ACV. – Stacy Ahmad, La Crosse, WI

Praises for Apple Cider Vinegar & The Bragg Healthy Lifestyle

I've had a fungi infection on my legs for years. I had been to doctors and dermatologists across the country, used $200 tubes of medicine, etc. to no avail. Recently I went to another local doctor and asked for anti fungi medication and he told me he really thought it was staph and talked me into another round of antibiotics . . . long story short the infection exploded and I was desperate! I have been reading and using Bragg products for years and found in your ACV book the cure!!! I am now 90% cured and feel better than ever!!! God Bless You!! As a Christian I am to take care of my temple, my body and you guys are a vital part. I am forever grateful. Blessings. – Jonathan Henson, Sherwood, AK

Many Blessings to you. I have been using your ACV with great success. My sinuses and lungs have cleared up. No more excess mucus, my head is clear and I have lost weight and feel naturally more happy. ACV is more effective than any combination of any herbs I have used in the past and is so affordable. Everyone should add this healthy remedy to their diet. It will add joy and years to anyone's life. – Mahashakti Das, Woodland Hills, CA

The Bragg Healthy Lifestyle, vinegar drink and brisk walking (3x daily) 20 minutes after meals, helped eliminate my diabetes! My whole body, circulation, feet, eyes have all improved. Thank you, may God continue to bless your Crusade. – John Risk, Santee, CA

I have been using your Organic Raw Apple Cider Vinegar with the "Mother" enzyme for 6 weeks . . . since then my joint aches and pains have reduced significantly. I breathe better and my general energy is up. Thanks. – Bob Tyler, West Palm Beach, FL

I have to start off by telling you and everyone else how amazingly delicious the ACV "cocktail" is! I had my first drink recently and I am in awe of the results. I was in a bad car accident and have had all kinds of physical injuries. One of them being terrible heartburn and nothing helped. Almost immediately after drinking the ACV my heartburn literally disappeared! I was able to sleep through the night. Thank you and may God bless you!– Christina Holland, Justin,TX

Food just isn't food in our house without Bragg Liquid Aminos. How can this amazing liquid make everything taste better than it naturally does? It's pure magic. Thanks to Paul and Patricia. – Adam Robinson, Portland, OR

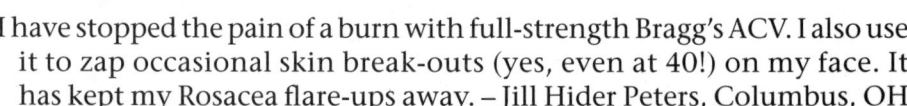

I have stopped the pain of a burn with full-strength Bragg's ACV. I also use it to zap occasional skin break-outs (yes, even at 40!) on my face. It has kept my Rosacea flare-ups away. – Jill Hider Peters, Columbus, OH

Praises for Apple Cider Vinegar & The Bragg Healthy Lifestyle

If I had to give up everything health related and keep only one item, Bragg ACV would be the one. At 35 years old, I felt like 95. I could hardly get through a day without going to bed in the afternoon. I tried everything and nothing helped. My wife's Grandpa "took an ACV nip" every morning and lived a long and active life, despite having smoked for a large part of his life. I also remember my Great Nana doing it. I tried it and in no time started feeling healthier and stronger! I am almost 37 now and have not been sick in over a year. I tell everyone about Bragg ACV and have given over 20 bottles away to family and friends. Thank You!!! Dave Streen, Williams Bay, WI

In Love – Promise Yourself

Promise yourself to be so strong that nothing
can disturb your peace of mind.

To talk Health, Happiness and Prosperity
to every person you meet.

To make all your friends feel that there is
something special in them.

To look at the sunny side of everything and
make your optimism come true.

To think only of the best, to work only for the best
and expect only the best.

To be just as enthusiastic about the success of
others as you are about your own.

To forget the mistakes of the past and press on
to the greater achievements of the future.

To be too large for worry, too noble for anger,
too strong for fear and too happy to permit
the presence of trouble and unhappiness.

To give so much time to the improvement of yourself
that you have no time to criticize others.

To wear a cheerful countenance at all times and
give every living creature you meet a smile.

Christian D. Larson

Deeds of kindness, smiles and little words of love and thanks help to make people and earth happy, like the Heaven above. – Julia Carney

HEALTH DREAM WITH NEW HEALTH VISION

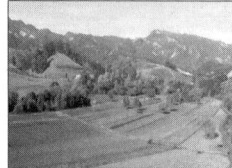 The Bragg Health Institute is located on a beautiful 120 acre Campus and Organic Farm on the coast of Santa Barbara, California. Patricia Bragg and the Directors of Bragg Health Institute have designated this as the future site of the greatest living tribute and memorial to the life of Paul C. Bragg. The new Bragg Center will become a world center for organic and healthy lifestyle education and research. (See the *Mission, Purpose and Vision for the Future* video on *www.bragghealthinstitute.org*)

You can also be part of Paul Bragg's lasting legacy by having your name permanently inscribed upon one of the educational nature walks or inspirational walls that will enhance the natural beauty of the Bragg Health Institute Campus and Organic Farm. Or you may want to have your name inscribed in the Grand Entrance or one of the rooms in the Bragg Memorial Library or Health Education Center. Your name can be part of your own legacy, as you will be recognized for generations to come as a great Health Crusader because of your special financial support of this wonderful project. When thousands of visitors see your name each year, they will know that you helped make a difference in the world.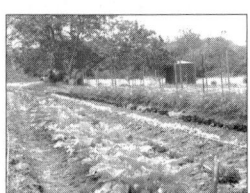

Some of the Special Projects for the new Bragg Health Center:

- Paul C. Bragg Memorial Library
- Organic Medicinal Herb Gardens
- Paul Bragg Memorial Rose Gardens
- Bragg Healthy Lifestyle videos & DVDs
- Healthy Cuisine Demo Kitchen

- Health Education Center
- Organic Teaching Gardens
- Bragg Nature & Farm Walks
- Bragg Health Museum
- Special Events & Programs

— — — — — — — —*MAKE COPY AND MAIL, FAX OR EMAIL* — — — — — — — —

YES! I would like to help support Bragg Health Crusades by making a contribution to the Bragg Health Institute, a 501(c)3 non-profit foundation. Your contributions are tax deductible.

❏ Enclosed is my tax-deductible gift of $_____ ○ CHECK ○ VISA ○ MC ○ Discover

❏ Please send me info on where my name can be permanently inscribed at the Bragg Center.

Credit Card Number:_____ Card Expires: _____ / _____
month / year

Signature:_____

• _____
Name

• _____ • _____
Address   **Apt. No.**

• _____ • _____ • _____
City   **State**   **Zip**

• (_____) • _____
Phone   **e-mail**

*If giving by check, please make check payable to: **Bragg Health Institute***
Mail To: Box 7, Santa Barbara, CA 93102 USA • (805) 968-1020

 For more info check out our web: www.bragghealthinstitute.org
Spreading health worldwide since 1912

BRAGG "HOW-TO, SELF-HEALTH" BOOKS

Authored by America's First Family of Health

Live Longer – Healthier – Stronger Self-Improvement Library

Qty.	BRAGG Book Titles Health Science ISBN: 978- 0-87790	Price	$ Total
	10 BRAGG Book Offer – Get Healthy, Live Longer Special – plus Free S&H ..only 89.00		
	(Please see next 2 pages for book descriptions)		
	Apple Cider Vinegar Miracle Health System – *(over 8 million in print)*	9.95	
	Back Fitness Program – For Pain-Free, Strong, Healthy Back	9.95	
	Bragg Healthy Lifestyle – Vital Living to 120 (formerly Toxicless Diet)	9.95	
	Build Powerful Nerve Force – Increase Energy, Eliminate Fatigue, Stress, Anger, Anxiety	11.95	
	Build Strong Healthy Feet – Banish Aches & Pains, Dr Scholl said "it's the best"	8.95	
	Healthy Heart – Keep Your Heart & Cardiovascular Healthy & Fit at any age	11.95	
	The Miracle of Fasting – Bragg Bible of Health, Physical Rejuvenation & Longevity ..	11.95	
	Super Power Breathing – for Super Energy, Longevity, & Heal Asthma, Allergies	11.95	
	Water, The Shocking Truth – That Can Save Your Life - Learn safest water to drink ...	8.95	
	Vegetarian Health Recipes – 700 Delicious, Nutritious, Healthy Recipes	13.95	
	BRAGG DVD – Enjoy BRAGG History, Lectures, Exercise Class, etc. ....only 7.95		

TOTAL COPIES	Books also available as E-books - see bragg.com Due to printing/paper costs, prices subject to change without notice.	**TOTAL BOOKS** $

Books Only: CA Residents add 8.75% tax

Please Specify: ☐ Check ☐ Money Order ☐ Credit Card

(S&H) Shipping & Handling

Charge To: ➤ ☐ Visa ☐ Master Card ☐ Discover

Month Year

VISA MasterCard DISCOVER

Card Expires

CVV #: _____

Credit Card Number

_____

Signature

(USA Funds Only)
TOTAL BOOKS $.

USA Shipping	Please add $5 first book, $1 each additional book USA retail book orders over $50 add $7 only
International Shipping	Canada add $11 for first book. $1.50 each additional book. All other Int'l. orders add $13. $1.50 each additional book

BOF 310

Name _____

Address _____ Apt. No. _____

City _____ State _____ Zip _____

Phone ( ) _____ e-mail _____

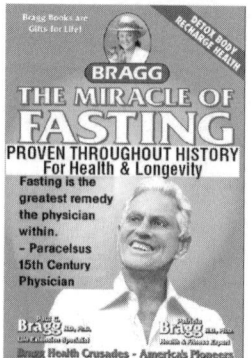
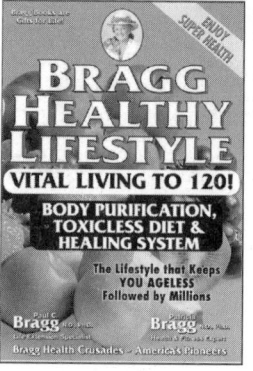
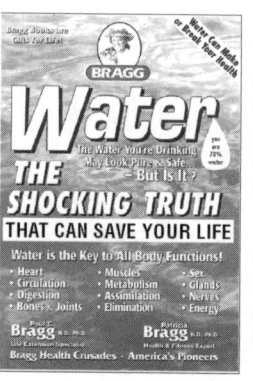
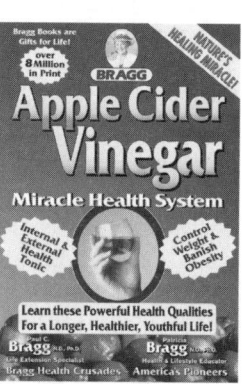
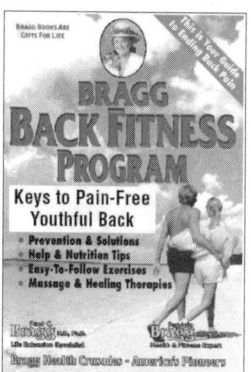
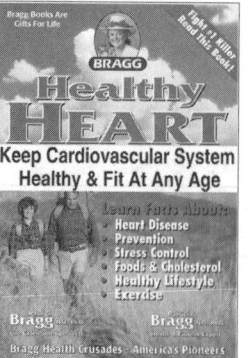
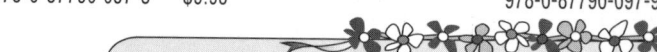

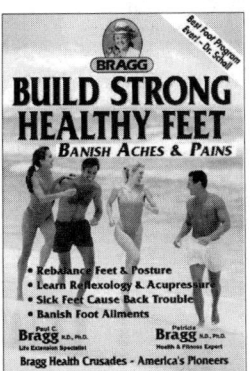
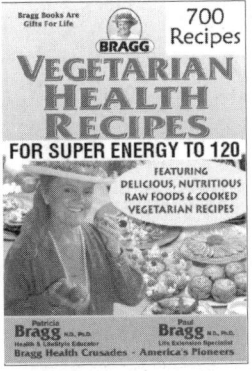
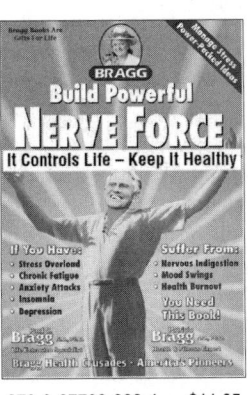
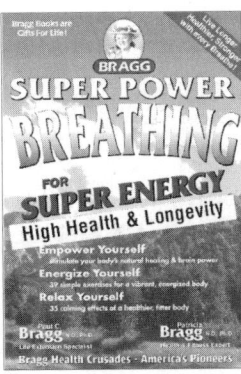

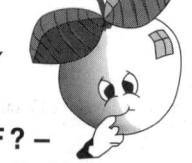
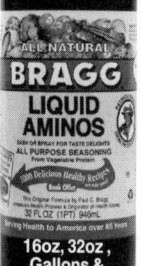
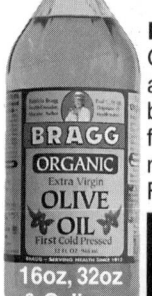

BRAGG ORGANIC APPLE CIDER VINEGAR

SIZE	PRICE	UPS SHIPPING & HANDLING For USA	$ Amount
16 oz.	$ 3.29 each	S/H – Please add $9. for 1st bottle and $1.50 each additional bottle	•
16 oz.	$ 36.00 Special Case /12	S/H Cost by Time Zone: CA $12. PST/MST $14. CST $22. EST $25	•
32 oz.	$ 5.29 each	S/H – Please add $10. for 1st bottle – $2. each additional bottle	•
32 oz.	$ 58.00 Special Case /12	S/H Cost by Time Zone: CA $17. PST/MST $20. CST $35. EST $38	•
1 gal.	$ 16.49 each	S/H – 1st bottle: CA $9. PST/MST $10. CST $13. EST $15 – $6. each add'l bottle	•
1 gal.	$ 57.00 Special Case /4	S/H Cost by Time Zone: CA $17. PST/MST $20. CST $34. EST $37	•

BRAGG Vinegar is a food and not taxable

BRAGG VINEGAR	$ •
(S&H) Shipping & Handling	•
TOTAL	$ •

BRAGG LIQUID AMINOS

SIZE	PRICE	UPS SHIPPING & HANDLING For USA	$ Amount
6 oz.	$ 3.59 each	S/H – Please add $9. for 1st 3 bottles – $1.50 each additional bottle	•
6 oz.	$ 78.00 Special Case /24	S/H Cost by Time Zone: CA $10. PST/MST $11. CST $17. EST $19	•
16 oz.	$ 4.69 each	S/H – Please add $9. for 1st bottle – $1.50 each additional bottle	•
16 oz.	$ 51.00 Special Case /12	S/H Cost by Time Zone: CA $12. PST/MST $14. CST $22. EST $25	•
32 oz.	$ 7.69 each	S/H – Please add $9. for 1st bottle and $2. each additional bottle	•
32 oz.	$ 84.00 Special Case /12	S/H Cost by Time Zone: CA $17. PST/MST $20. CST $35. EST $38	•
1 gal.	$ 28.39 each	S/H – 1st bottle: CA $10. PST/MST $10. CST $13. EST $15 – $6. each add'l bottle	•
1 gal.	$ 99.00 Special Case /4	S/H Cost by Time Zone: CA $17. PST/MST $20. CST $34. EST $37	•

BRAGG Aminos & Olive Oil are foods and not taxable

BRAGG AMINOS	$ •
(S&H) Shipping & Handling	•
TOTAL	$ •

BRAGG ORGANIC OLIVE OIL

SIZE	PRICE	UPS SHIPPING & HANDLING For USA	$ Amount
16 oz.	$ 10.99 each	S/H – Please add $9. for 1st bottle – $1.50 each additional bottle	•
16 oz.	$ 120.00 Special Case /12	S/H Cost by Time Zone: CA $12. PST/MST $14. CST $22. EST $25	•
32 oz.	$ 17.89 each	S/H – Please add $10. for 1st bottle and $2. each additional bottle	•
32 oz.	$ 196.00 Special Case /12	S/H Cost by Time Zone: CA $17. PST/MST $20. CST $35. EST $38	•
1 gal.	$ 62.69 each	S/H – 1st bottle: CA $10. PST/MST $10. CST $13. EST $15 – $6. each add'l bottle	•
1 gal.	$ 219.00 Special Case /4	S/H Cost by Time Zone: CA $17. PST/MST $20. CST $34. EST $37	•

Please Specify: ☐ Check ☐ Money Order ☐ Cash
Charge to: ☐ Visa ☐ Master Card ☐ Discover

Credit Card
Number:_____

Card Expires: _____ / _____
month / year

BRAGG OLIVE OIL	$ •
(S&H) Shipping & Handling	•
TOTAL	$ •

VISA
MasterCard
DISCOVER

Signature:_____

Business office calls (805) 968-1020. We accept MasterCard, Discover & VISA phone orders. Please prepare order using order form. It speeds your call and serves as order record. Hours: 8 to 4 pm Pacific Time, Monday thru Thursday.

• Visit our Web: www.bragg.com • e-mail: bragg @ bragg.com

CREDIT CARD ORDERS
CALL (800) 446-1990
OR FAX (805) 968-1001

BOF 310

Mail to: **HEALTH SCIENCE, Box 7, Santa Barbara, CA 93102 USA**
Please Print or Type – Be sure to give street & house number to facilitate delivery.

Name _____

Address _____ Apt. No. _____

City _____ State _____ Zip _____

Phone (___) _____ e-mail _____

Bragg Health Products available most Health Stores & Grocery Health Depts Nationwide

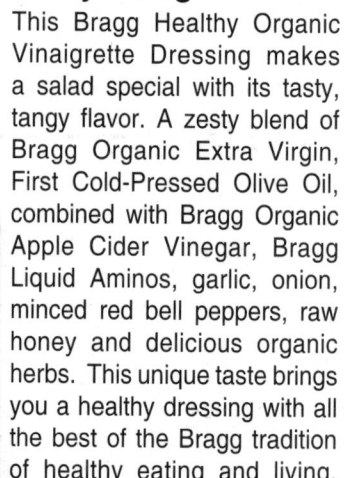
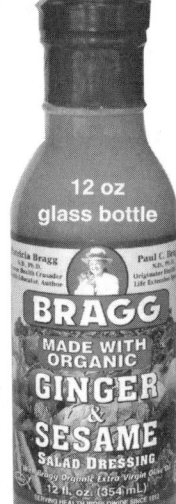
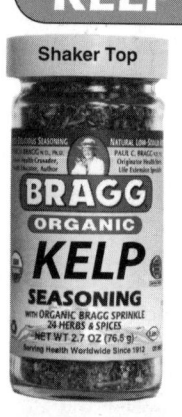
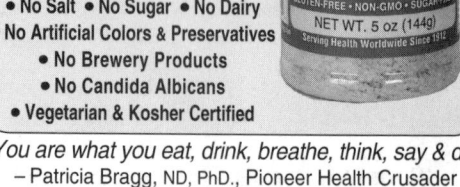

BRAGG SPRINKLE – 24 Herbs & Spices Seasoning

SIZE	PRICE		UPS SHIPPING & HANDLING For USA	$	Amount
1.5 oz.	$ 4.69	each	S/H – Please add $9. for 1st 3 bottles and $1. each additional bottle		.
1.5 oz.	$ 51.00	Special Case /12	S/H Cost by Time Zone: CA $9. PST/MST $9. CST $10. EST $12.		.
			BRAGG SPRINKLE	$	.
BRAGG Sprinkle Seasoning is a food and not taxable			(S&H) Shipping & Handling		.
			TOTAL	$	.

BRAGG ORGANIC SEA KELP

SIZE	PRICE		UPS SHIPPING & HANDLING For USA	$	Amount
2.7 oz.	$ 4.69	each	S/H – Please add $9. for 1st 3 bottles and $1. each additional bottle		.
2.7 oz.	$ 51.00	Special Case /12	S/H Cost by Time Zone: CA $9. PST/MST $9. CST $10. EST $12.		.
			BRAGG KELP	$	.
BRAGG Kelp Seasoning is a food and not taxable			(S&H) Shipping & Handling		.
			TOTAL	$	.

BRAGG NUTRITIONAL YEAST

SIZE	PRICE		UPS SHIPPING & HANDLING For USA	$	Amount
4.5 oz.	$ 6.29	each	S/H – Please add $9. for 1st 3 bottles and $1. each additional bottle		.
4.5 oz.	$ 69.00	Special Case /12	S/H Cost by Time Zone: CA $9. PST/MST $9. CST $10. EST $12.		.
			BRAGG YEAST		
BRAGG Nutritional Yeast Seasoning is a food and not taxable			(S&H) Shipping & Handling		.
			TOTAL	$	.

BRAGG SALAD DRESSINGS

SIZE	PRICE		UPS SHIPPING & HANDLING For USA	$	Amount
✳ BRAGG GINGER & SESAME SALAD DRESSING					
12 oz.	$ 5.49	each	S/H – Please add $9. for 1st bottle and $1.25 each additional bottle		.
12 oz.	$ 60.00	Special Case /12	S/H Cost by Time Zone: CA $11. PST/MST $12. CST $19. EST $22		.
✳ BRAGG ORGANIC VINAIGRETTE SALAD DRESSING					
12 oz.	$ 5.49	each	S/H – Please add $9. for 1st bottle and $1.25 each additional bottle		.
12 oz.	$ 60.00	Special Case /12	S/H Cost by Time Zone: CA $11. PST/MST $12. CST $19. EST $22		.
BRAGG Salad Dressings are foods and not taxable			BRAGG SALAD DRESSINGS	$	.
			(S&H) Shipping & Handling		.
			TOTAL	$	.

Payment Method:

☐ Check ☐ Money Order ☐ Cash

Charge To: ☐ Visa ☐ Master Card ☐ Discover

Credit Card Number:_____

Card Expires:_____ / _____
month / year

Signature:_____

Business office calls (805) 968-1020. We accept MasterCard, Discover & VISA phone orders. Please prepare order using order form. It speeds your call and serves as order record. Hours: 8 to 4 pm Pacific Time, Monday thru Thursday. • Visit our Web: www.bragg.com • e-mail: bragg @ bragg.com

CREDIT CARD ORDERS
CALL (800) 446-1990
OR FAX (805) 968-1001

BOF 310

Mail to: **HEALTH SCIENCE, Box 7, Santa Barbara, CA 93102 USA**

Please Print or Type – Be sure to give street & house number to facilitate delivery.

Name _____

Address _____ Apt. No. _____

City _____ State _____ Zip _____

(___) _____ e-mail _____
Phone

Bragg Products available most Health Stores & Grocery Health Depts Nationwide

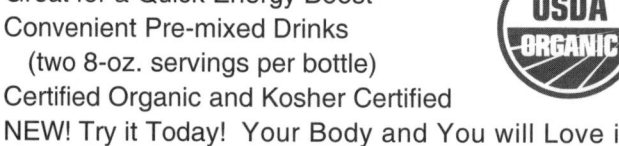
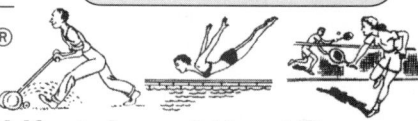

BRAGG ORGANIC APPLE CIDER VINEGAR DRINKS

DRINK FLAVORS	SIZE	PRICE	QTY	CASE PRICE	QTY	$	Amount
Original Apple Cider Vinegar & Honey - 16 oz	$2.19			$24.00			.
ACV with Ginger - Spice - 16 oz	$2.19			$24.00			.
ACV with Apple - Cinnamon - 16 oz	$2.19			$24.00			.
ACV with Concord Grape - Acai - 16 oz	$2.19			$24.00			.

BRAGG APPLE CIDER VINEGAR DRINKS are Foods and are not taxable

BRAGG VINEGAR DRINK $.

(S&H) Shipping & Handling .

SHIPPING CHART FOR ACV DRINKS ↖

TOTAL $.

Number of bottles	CA	PST/MST	CST	EST
1-2 bottles	$8.00	$8.00	$9.00	$12.00
3-4 bottles	$8.00	$9.00	$11.00	$13.00
5-6 bottles	$9.00	$9.00	$13.00	$15.00
7-12 bottles	$11.00	$13.00	$21.00	$24.00
Special Case/12	$11.00	$13.00	$21.00	$24.00

BRAGGZYME – Systemic Enzymes

SIZE	PRICE	UPS SHIPPING & HANDLING For USA	$	Amount
120 cap	$ 43.95 each	S/H – Please add $9. for 1st 3 bottles and $1. each additional bottle		.
120 cap	$ 483.00 Special Case/12	S/H Cost by Time Zone: CA $9. PST/MST $10. CST $11. EST $12.		.

on Braggzyme CA Residents only pay tax

for BRAGGZYME only CA Residents add 8.75% TAX $.

(S&H) Shipping & Handling .

TOTAL $.

Payment Method:

☐ Check ☐ Money Order ☐ Cash

Charge To: ☐ Visa ☐ Master Card ☐ Discover

Credit Card Number:_____

Card Expires:_____ month / year

Signature:_____

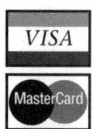

Business office calls (805) 968-1020
We accept MasterCard, Discover & VISA
Phone orders please prepare order using order forms,
as it speeds up your call and serves as your order record.
Hours: 8 to 4 pm Pacific Time, Monday thru Thursday.
• Visit Web: www.bragg.com • e-mail: bragg @ bragg.com

CREDIT CARD ORDERS CALL:
(800) 446-1990
OR FAX (805) 968-1001

BOF 310

Mail to: **HEALTH SCIENCE, Box 7, Santa Barbara, CA 93102 USA**
Please Print or Type – Be sure to give street & house number to facilitate delivery.

Name _____

Address _____ Apt. No. _____

City _____ State _____ Zip _____

Phone ( ) _____ e-mail _____

Bragg Products available most Health Stores & Grocery Health Depts Nationwide

– Make copies when needed for mailing in. –

Send for Free Health Bulletins

Patricia Bragg wants to keep in touch with you, your relatives and friends about the latest Health, Nutrition, Exercise and Longevity Discoveries. Please enclose one stamp for each USA name listed. Foreign listings send postal reply coupons.

With Blessings of Health, Peace and Thanks

Please make copy, then print clearly and mail to: *Patricia*

BRAGG HEALTH CRUSADES, Box 7, Santa Barbara, CA 93102

● Name

● Address ● Apt. No.

● City ● State ● Zip

● Phone ( ) ● e-mail

● Name

● Address ● Apt. No.

● City ● State ● Zip

● Phone ( ) ● e-mail

● Name

● Address ● Apt. No.

● City ● State ● Zip

● Phone ( ) ● e-mail

● Name

● Address ● Apt. No.

● City ● State ● Zip

● Phone ( ) ● e-mail

● Name

● Address ● Apt. No.

● City ● State ● Zip

● Phone ( ) ● e-mail

Bragg Health Crusades spreading health worldwide since 1912

PATRICIA BRAGG, N.D., Ph.D.
Health Crusader & Angel of Health & Healing

Author, Lecturer, Nutritionist, Health & Lifestyle Educator to World Leaders, Hollywood Stars, Singers, Athletes, etc. & Millions.

Patricia is a 100% dedicated health crusader with a passion like her father, Paul C. Bragg, world renowned health authority. Patricia has won international fame on her own in this field. She conducts Bragg Health and Fitness Seminars for Conventions and Women's, Men's, Youth and Church Groups around the world and promotes Bragg Healthy Lifestyle Living and "How-To, Self-Health" Books on Radio and TV Talk Shows throughout the English-speaking world. Consultants to Presidents and Royalty, to Stars of Stage, Screen and TV and to Champion Athletes, Patricia and her father co-authored The Bragg Health Library of Instructive, Inspiring Books that promote a healthier lifestyle, for a long, healthy, happy life.

Patricia herself is the symbol of health, perpetual youthfulness and radiant, feminine energy. She is a living and sparkling example of her and her father's healthy lifestyle precepts and this she loves sharing world-wide.

A fifth-generation Californian on her mother's side, Patricia was reared by The Bragg Natural Health Method from infancy. In school, she not only excelled in athletics, but also won honors for her studies and her counseling. She is an accomplished musician and dancer . . . as well as tennis player and mountain climber . . . and the youngest woman ever to be granted a U.S. Patent. Patricia is a popular gifted Health Teacher and a dynamic, in-demand Talk Show Guest on Radio and TV where she regularly spreads the simple, easy-to-follow Bragg Healthy Lifestyle for everyone of all ages.

Man's body is his vehicle through life, his earthly temple . . . and the Creator wants us filled with joy & health for a long fruitful life. The Bragg Crusades of Health and Fitness (3 John 2) has carried her around the world over 20 times – spreading physical, emotional, mental and spiritual health and joy. Health is our birthright and Patricia teaches how to prevent the destruction of our health from man-made wrong lifestyle habits of living.

Patricia's been a Health Consultant to American Presidents, British Royalty, to Champion Triathletes and Betty Cuthbert, Australia's "Golden Girl," (16 world records and 4 Olympic track gold medals) and New Zealand's Olympic Track and Triathlete Star, Allison Roe. Among those who come to her for advice are some of Hollywood's top Stars from Clint Eastwood to the ever-youthful singing group, The Beach Boys and their families, Singing Stars of the Metropolitan Opera and top Ballet Stars. Patricia's message is of world-wide appeal to people of all ages, nationalities and walks-of-life. Those who follow The Bragg Healthy Lifestyle and attend the Bragg Crusades world-wide are living testimonials . . . like ageless, super athlete, Jack LaLanne, who at age 15 went from sickness to Total Fitness and Health!

Patricia inspires you to Renew, Rejuvenate and Revitalize your life with "The Bragg Healthy Lifestyle" Books and Health Crusades worldwide. Millions have benefitted from these life-changing events with a longer, healthier and happier life! She loves to share with your community, organization, church groups, etc. Also, she is a perfect radio and TV talk show guest to spread the message of healthy lifestyle living. See and hear Patricia on the web: bragg.com
For radio interview & lecture requests write or e-mail: **patricia@bragg.com**
BRAGG HEALTH CRUSADES, BOX 7, SANTA BARBARA, CA 93102, USA